Disease-Based Physical Examination

Editor

PAUL ARONOWITZ

MEDICAL CLINICS OF NORTH AMERICA

www.medical.theclinics.com

Consulting Editor
JACK ENDE

May 2022 • Volume 106 • Number 3

ELSEVIER

1600 John F. Kennedy Boulevard ● Suite 1800 ● Philadelphia, Pennsylvania, 19103-2899

http://www.theclinics.com

MEDICAL CLINICS OF NORTH AMERICA Volume 106, Number 3
May 2022 ISSN 0025-7125, ISBN-13: 978-0-323-91998-2

Editor: Katerina Heidhausen
Developmental Editor: Arlene Campos

Medical Clinics of North America (ISSN 0025-7125) is published bimonthly by Elsevier Inc., 360 Park Avenue South, New York, NY 10010-1710. Months of publication are January, March, May, July, September, and November. Business and editorial offices: 1600 John F. Kennedy Boulevard, Suite 1800, Philadelphia, PA 19103-2899. Periodicals postage paid at New York, NY, and additional mailing offices. Subscription prices are USD $316.00 per year (US individuals), $956.00 per year (US institutions), $100.00 per year (US Students), $396.00 per year (Canadian individuals), $1,004.00 per year (Canadian institutions), $200.00 per year for (foreign students), $100.00 per year for (Canadian students), $439.00 per year (foreign individuals), and $1,004.00 per year (foreign institutions). To receive student/resident rate, orders must be accompanied by name of affiliated institution, date of term, and the signature of program/residency coordinator on institution letterhead. Orders will be billed at individual rate until proof of status is received. Foreign air speed delivery is included in all Clinics' subscription prices. All prices are subject to change without notice. **POSTMASTER:** Send address changes to *Medical Clinics of North America*, Elsevier Health Sciences Division, Subscription Customer Service, 3251 Riverport Lane, Maryland Heights, MO 63043. **Customer Service: Telephone: 1-800-654-2452** (U.S. and Canada); **1-314-447-8871** (outside U.S. and Canada). **Fax: 314-447-8029. E-mail: journalscustomerserviceusa@elsevier.com** (for print support); **journalsonlinesupport-usa@elsevier.com** (for online support).

Reprints. For copies of 100 or more of articles in this publication, please contact the Commercial Reprints Department, Elsevier Inc., 360 Park Avenue South, New York, NY 10010-1710. Tel.: 212-633-3874; Fax: 212-633-3820; E-mail: reprints@elsevier.com.

Medical Clinics of North America is also published in Spanish by McGraw-Hill Interamericana Editores S. A., P.O. Box 5-237, 06500 Mexico, D.F., Mexico.

Medical Clinics of North America is covered in *MEDLINE/PubMed (Index Medicus), Current Contents, ASCA, Excerpta Medica, Science Citation Index,* and *ISI/BIOMED.*

PROGRAM OBJECTIVE
The goal of the *Medical Clinics of North America* is to keep practicing physicians up to date with current clinical practice by providing timely articles reviewing the state of the art in patient care.

TARGET AUDIENCE
All practicing physicians and other healthcare professionals.

LEARNING OBJECTIVES
Upon completion of this activity, participants will be able to:
1. Review the characteristics and clinical presentation of common cancers, pulmonary, metabolic, endocrine, cardiac, neurologic, hemodynamic, and infectious disorders.
2. Explain the benefits of the physical assessment in gathering patient health data to guide in the development of the diagnosis, prognosis, and treatment strategies for common health disorders.
3. Discuss the role of the physical assessment as a tool in diagnosing, treating, and assessment of treatment response in common health disorders.

ACCREDITATION
The Elsevier Office of Continuing Medical Education (EOCME) is accredited by the Accreditation Council for Continuing Medical Education (ACCME) to provide continuing medical education for physicians.

The EOCME designates this journal-based CME activity for a maximum of 13 *AMA PRA Category 1 Credit*(s)™. Physicians should claim only the credit commensurate with the extent of their participation in the activity.

All other healthcare professionals requesting continuing education credit for this enduring material will be issued a certificate of participation.

DISCLOSURE OF CONFLICTS OF INTEREST
The EOCME assesses conflict of interest with its instructors, faculty, planners, and other individuals who are in a position to control the content of CME activities. All relevant conflicts of interest that are identified are thoroughly vetted by EOCME for fair balance, scientific objectivity, and patient care recommendations. EOCME is committed to providing its learners with CME activities that promote improvements or quality in healthcare and not a specific proprietary business or a commercial interest.

The planning committee, staff, authors, and editors listed below have identified no financial relationships or relationships to products or devices they or their spouse/life partner have with commercial interest related to the content of this CME activity:
Reeni Ann Abraham, MD; Sonia Ananthakrishnan, MD; Paul Aronowitz, MD, MACP; Lisa Bernstein, MD, FACP; Stephanie Kaye Brinker, MD; Jennifer Chen, MD; Heather E. Harrell, MD; Mark Henderson, MD, MACP; Sharad Jain, MD; Craig R Keenan, MD, FACP; Kristen D. Kelley, MD, MAS; Christopher L Knight, MD; John Landefeld, MD, MS; Aamir Malik, MBBS; Jason D Napolitano, MD, FACP; Merlin Packiam; Deepti Pujare, MD; Dana Sheely, MD; Kim Tartaglia, MD; Doreen Thomas-Payne, MSN, BSN, RN, PMHNP-BC; Melody Tran-Reina, MD; Donna M Williams, MD; Rachel Wilson, DO; Daniel Winkel, MD; Ashleigh EH Wright, MD

UNAPPROVED/OFF-LABEL USE DISCLOSURE
The EOCME requires CME faculty to disclose to the participants:
1. When products or procedures being discussed are off-label, unlabelled, experimental, and/or investigational (not US Food and Drug Administration [FDA] approved); and
2. Any limitations on the information presented, such as data that are preliminary or that represent ongoing research, interim analyses, and/or unsupported opinions. Faculty may discuss information about pharmaceutical agents that is outside of FDA-approved labelling. This information is intended solely for CME and is not intended to promote off-label use of these medications. If you have any questions, contact the medical affairs department of the manufacturer for the most recent prescribing information.

TO ENROLL
To enroll in the *Medical Clinics of North America* Continuing Medical Education program, call customer service at 1-800-654-2452 or sign up online at http://www.theclinics.com/home/cme. The CME program is available to subscribers for an additional annual fee of USD 324.00.

METHOD OF PARTICIPATION

In order to claim credit, participants must complete the following;

1. Complete enrolment as indicated above.
2. Read the activity.
3. Complete the CME Test and Evaluation. Participants must achieve a score of 70% on the test. All CME Tests and Evaluations must be completed online.

CME INQUIRIES/SPECIAL NEEDS

For all CME inquiries or special needs, please contact elsevierCME@elsevier.com.

FORTHCOMING ISSUES

July 2022
**Communication Skills and Challenges in
Medical Practice**
Heather Hofmann, *Editor*

September 2022
**Nutrition in the Practice of Medicine: A
Practical Approach**
David S Seres, *Editor*

November 2022
Clinical Psychiatry
Leo Sher, *Editor*

RECENT ISSUES

March 2022
Update in Preventive Cardiology
Douglas S. Jacoby, *Editor*

January 2022
Substance Use Disorders
Melissa B. Weimer, *Editor*

November 2021
Update in Endocrinology
Silvio Inzucchi and Elizabeth H. Holt,
Editors

MEDICAL CLINICS OF NORTH AMERICA

CLINICS

Contributors

CONSULTING EDITOR

JACK ENDE, MD, MACP
The Schaeffer Professor of Medicine, Perelman School of Medicine, University of Pennsylvania, Philadelphia, Pennsylvania

EDITOR

PAUL ARONOWITZ, MD, MACP
Health Sciences Clinical Professor of Medicine, Department of Medicine, University of California, Davis School of Medicine, Sacramento, California

AUTHORS

REENI ANN ABRAHAM, MD
Associate Professor, Division of General Internal Medicine, UT Southwestern Medical Center, Dallas, Texas

SONIA ANANTHAKRISHNAN, MD
Assistant Professor of Medicine, Boston University School of Medicine/Boston Medical Center, Section of Endocrinology, Diabetes and Nutrition, Boston, Massachusetts

PAUL ARONOWITZ, MD, MACP
Health Sciences Clinical Professor of Medicine, Department of Medicine, University of California, Davis School of Medicine, Sacramento, California

LISA BERNSTEIN, MD, FACP
Professor, Department of Medicine, Division of General Internal Medicine, Emory University School of Medicine, Atlanta, Georgia

STEPHANIE KAYE BRINKER, MD
Associate Professor, Division of General Internal Medicine, UT Southwestern Medical Center, Dallas, Texas

JENNIFER CHEN, MD
Health Sciences Assistant Clinical Professor of Medicine, Department of Internal Medicine, University of California, Davis, Sacramento, California

HEATHER E. HARRELL, MD
Professor of Internal Medicine, University of Florida, Gainesville, Florida

MARK HENDERSON, MD MACP
Professor and Vice Chair for Education, Department of Internal Medicine, University of California, Davis School of Medicine, Sacramento, California

SHARAD JAIN, MD
Professor of Medicine, Assistant Dean for Student Affairs, University of California, Davis School of Medicine, Sacramento, California

CRAIG R. KEENAN, MD, FACP
Professor of Medicine, Internal Medicine Residency Program Director, University of California, Davis School of Medicine, Sacramento, California

KRISTEN D. KELLEY, MD, MAS
Associate Physician, Division of General Internal Medicine, UC Davis Heath, Sacramento, California

CHRISTOPHER L. KNIGHT, MD
Associate Professor of Medicine, University of Washington, Seattle, Washington

JOHN LANDEFELD, MD MS
Assistant Clinical Professor, Department of Internal Medicine, University of California, Davis School of Medicine, Sacramento, California

AAMIR MALIK, MBBS
Fellow in Endocrinology, Boston University School of Medicine/Boston Medical Center, Section of Endocrinology, Diabetes and Nutrition, Boston, Massachusetts

JASON D. NAPOLITANO, MD
Professor of Clinical Medicine, David Geffen School of Medicine at UCLA, Los Angeles, California

DEEPTI PUJARE, MD
Division of Endocrinology, Diabetes and Metabolism, University of California, Davis, Sacramento, California

DANA SHEELY, MD
Associate Professor, Division of Endocrinology, Diabetes and Metabolism, University of California, Davis, Sacramento, California

KIM TARTAGLIA, MD
Professor of Clinical Medicine and Pediatrics, Department of Internal Medicine, The Ohio State University College of Medicine, Columbus, Ohio

MELODY TRAN-REINA, MD
Assistant Clinical Professor, Department of Internal Medicine, University of California, Davis School of Medicine, Sacramento, California

DONNA M. WILLIAMS, MD
Associate Professor, Section on General Internal Medicine, Wake Forest School of Medicine, Winston-Salem, North Carolina

RACHEL WILSON, DO
Assistant Clinical Professor, University of Wisconsin School of Medicine and Public Health, Madison, WI

DANIEL WINKEL, MD
Assistant Professor, Department of Neurology, Emory University School of Medicine, Atlanta, Georgia

ASHLEIGH E.H. WRIGHT, MD
Clinical Associate Professor of Internal Medicine, University of Florida, Gainesville, Florida

Contents

Kristen D. Kelley and Paul Aronowitz

Malignancy is the second leading cause of death in the United States, following heart disease. In most cancers, early detection is one of the most important factors in determining prognosis. As clinicians it is therefore important to be aware of potential clues of underlying malignancy on physical examination. Given the wide range of malignancies, and the heterogeneous nature of their presentations, this article is by no means exhaustive. Instead, it discusses in depth some of the more frequently encountered physical examination findings that may suggest malignancy. Specifically, it covers lymphadenopathy, cutaneous findings related to various cancers, and malignancy related thrombosis.

Reeni Ann Abraham and Stephanie Kaye Brinker

Performing a hypothesis-driven examination in patients with possible chronic obstructive pulmonary disease (COPD) is an important component of increasing the recognition and diagnosis of this avoidable and costly medical condition. Using known likelihood ratios for various physical examination maneuvers can be combined with known individual risk factors and symptoms to adjust a patient's post-test probability of having COPD and inform appropriate diagnostic work-up. Equally important is intentionality in history-taking and physical examination procedures for patients with known COPD to mitigate the decreased quality of life and mortality and to monitor response to treatment.

Rachel Wilson and Donna M. Williams

Cirrhosis is a chronic condition resulting from inflammation and fibrosis of the liver. Patients with cirrhosis may have a myriad of physical examination findings that reflect the severity of the underlying liver disease. Although many signs and symptoms related to cirrhosis are nonspecific, such as abdominal pain, nausea, and malaise, some findings are more specific and point to complications of liver disease. In this article, key physical findings in patients with cirrhosis, including hepatomegaly, splenomegaly, jaundice, ascites, encephalopathy, dilated abdominal wall veins, spider nevi, palmar erythema, and others, are discussed.

The physical examination of the patient with diabetes may have revealed findings that confirm the diagnosis, classify the type of diabetes, and begin to evaluate for the macro- and microvascular complications of diabetes and significant comorbid conditions. While screening for the diagnosis of diabetes occurs with assessment for abnormal blood glucose, given the high rates of morbidity and mortality associated with diabetes, utilization of the physical examination plays a key role in identifying patients at risk for the complications of diabetes. The discussion of elements of the physical examination relevant to the patient with diabetes, both type 1 and type 2, will be discussed in this article.

Many common endocrinopathies have classic physical examination findings that can help lead to the diagnosis and cause of disease. This article will discuss the common signs and symptoms seen in Cushing disease, adrenal insufficiency, hyperthyroidism, hypothyroidism, thyroid nodules, and polycystic ovary syndrome (PCOS). A knowledge of these findings and their corresponding diseases will help the clinician to develop a targeted examination for syndromes of excess or deficient cortisol, excess or deficient thyroid hormone, thyroid nodules, and PCOS.

Hypovolemia develops with the loss of extracellular fluid volume or blood. Rapidly identifying hypovolemia can be lifesaving. Indicators of hypovolemia on examination include supine or postural hypotension, increase in heart rate by 30 beats per minute or severe dizziness with standing, and a decrease in central venous pressure detected on visual inspection of the jugular venous pressure or ultrasound assessment of the inferior vena cava or internal jugular veins. Other findings with utility include a dry axilla and dry oral mucosa. With chronic anemia, hemodynamic changes detectable on examination may be minimal, as the body compensates by retaining extracellular volume.

Movement disorders are commonly encountered by the general practitioner and can be divided into two broad categories: hypokinetic and hyperkinetic. The former involves loss or slowing of movement, whereas the latter is characterized by excessive and involuntary movements. A careful history will guide the examiner to the appropriate category of movement disorders. As no laboratory test or radiologic study is confirmatory for these disorders, the diagnosis must be made clinically and the neurologic examination is indispensable. In this article, we discuss physical examination techniques that will help diagnose common movement disorders.

Foreword

For the Benefit of Us All

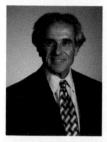

Jack Ende, MD, MACP
Consulting Editor

There are several reasons practicing clinicians should hold fast to their physical examination skills, and cutting costs is among the least important. Yes, the physical examination can focus a diagnostic workup and save costs. And, yes, the patients benefit from (and expect) a well-done physical examination. But most importantly, and rarely discussed, is the impact of the physical examination upon the clinician. That's right, the clinician.

As Guest Editor, Paul Aronowitz, ably explains, and as his carefully chosen authors beautifully illustrate, a well-done physical examination can be the difference between a diagnosis made and a diagnosis missed. Patients benefit; health care delivery becomes more cost-effective, and resources utilization improves. These reasons alone substantiate the importance of physical examination skills.

But here I also wish to underscore the benefits of the physical examination for the clinician, that is, the doctor, not the patient. Medicine is hard. Burnout is real. So many of our colleagues are frustrated, or worse. A major component of all this angst, I believe, is that we no longer feel like doctors. We went into our profession not to run patients through gauntlets of tests waiting for a diagnosis to emerge at the other end. I believe we went into medicine because we were captivated by physiology and pathophysiology, and how, using our eyes, ears, hands, and general powers of observation, we are able to figure out what is wrong with our patients.

I, for one, never feel more fulfilled as a clinician than when I can discover what my patient's problem is using physical examination. I am fortunate to practice general internal medicine and can test myself across a wide range of organ systems. I also take care of well patients, in whom unexpected physical examination findings can be critical, as was the recent discovery in the office of a pneumothorax in a patient with non-exertional chest pain; or in another patient who was found to have "wide open" mitral regurgitation presenting as a nocturnal cough. I take care of patients with known medical problems, heart failure, for instance, where physical examination has enabled me

Med Clin N Am 106 (2022) xiii–xiv
https://doi.org/10.1016/j.mcna.2022.02.005

to decide who needs further intervention or evaluation; or which of my patients with COPD might benefit from up-titrating inhalers. Now that we all have gained experience with telemedicine, I suspect we all appreciate, more now than ever before, the value of physical examination not only for the patient, but again, for the impact it can have on physician satisfaction.

When Dr Aronowitz and I began discussing this issue of *Medical Clinics of North America*, almost 1 year ago, we both knew we wanted to offer a resource for clinicians facing specific medical issues. Physical diagnosis can be empowering. I hope you agree.

Jack Ende, MD, MACP
The Schaeffer Professor of Medicine
Perelman School of Medicine of the
University of Pennsylvania
5033 West Gates Pavilion
3400 Spruce Street
Philadelphia, PA 19104, USA

E-mail address:
jack.ende@pennmedicine.upenn.edu

Preface

The Disease-Based Physical Examination

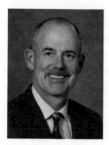

Paul Aronowitz, MD, MACP
Editor

Despite a decline in both the quality and the quantity of teaching of the physical examination in medical schools and postgraduate training programs over the past 4 decades, the physical examination remains a vital component of the patient assessment. Unlike most laboratory and radiologic tests, the physical examination provides immediate, often essential information at the patient bedside. Since the exam follows the history, it provides an opportunity to test hypotheses initially generated while the history is taken. For example, will a patient complaining of dyspnea, orthopnea, paroxysmal nocturnal dyspnea, and lower-extremity edema have an elevated jugular venous pulse, displaced cardiac point of maximal impulse, an S3 and crackles indicative of congestive heart failure? Will the patient suffering from alcoholism who presents reporting that her skin has turned yellow and that her pants no longer fit due to increased abdominal girth have dilated abdominal vessels, decreased body hair, and palmar erythema indicative of cirrhosis of the liver? The physical exam often also provides crucial information regarding response to therapy. Has the patient admitted to the hospital for erysipelas improved since being started on antibiotics? Has the jugular venous distension in the patient with congestive heart failure decreased after diuresis? Knowledge and skill at assessing disease-specific findings on the physical examination and, where possible, knowing and understanding the test characteristics of these findings elevate the clinician from novice data gatherer to master clinician.

In our health care systems that tend to elevate and reward frequent and sometimes unnecessary test ordering by providers who often don't feel confident in their own physical examination skills, acquiring and then maintaining disease-focused physical exam skills is difficult. A sense that technology, no matter the cost, is almost always better can lead to a sense of nihilism about the physical examination from the perspectives of both beginners and the experienced. Fifteen years ago, while working at a

Med Clin N Am 106 (2022) xv–xvii
https://doi.org/10.1016/j.mcna.2022.01.012
0025-7125/22/© 2022 Published by Elsevier Inc.

busy, urban hospital, I had consulted one of our best cardiologists—a clinician known to be highly skilled in the cardiac physical exam. I happened to be at the nursing station when he exited my patient's room.

"Can I borrow your stethoscope?" he asked me.

"What kind of a cardiologist does not carry a stethoscope?" I quipped.

"I stopped carrying it last year," he responded. "Now I mostly just order an Echocardiogram on all of my new patients, and I don't worry about listening to their hearts. " He was completely serious. Despite the years he had invested in building up his considerable skillset in the cardiac physical exam, it had become less time consuming and, from his perspective, higher yield to push a few buttons in the electronic medical record and order an echocardiogram. As depressing as this anecdote is, the counter to it is that I have rarely met a learner who wasn't interested in improving her physical examination skills and learning more about the art and history of physical diagnosis.

However, the era of bedside rounds, bedside presentations, and bedside physical examination has been supplanted by the electronic medical record and a golden age of radiology. Medical schools teach the physical examination, but it is mostly taught in state-of-the-art simulation centers on healthy standardized patients paid by the hour and devoid of significant physical findings. They are often taught to perform the exam in a rote fashion, not really knowing what they are looking, feeling, or listening for. It is good to know what is normal—clearly essential knowledge in order to be able to know what is abnormal—but this physical examination teaching often fails to continue into the setting of the hospital or clinic in the company of meaningful and authentic patients with real disease and physical exam abnormalities. The opportunity to compare and contrast normal with abnormal physical findings is not taught and cultivated, and so these skills wither, if they ever existed at all.

In the stressful and hectic work environments of modern clinics and hospitals, physical finding rounds—sometimes called "Discovery Rounds"—and bedside rounds have faded to practically nothing. The vast preponderance of attending rounds time is spent rounding in conference rooms or hallways and not at the bedsides of patients. A cardiac murmur or an extra heart sound is a recording heard in a classroom, not in a patient in the Cardiac Care Unit or the Emergency Department. When learners do come across patients with notable physical findings during their work, the findings are often missed, or the learner fails to have these findings corroborated by a clinician with adequate skill or confidence or because a clinician who possesses skill and confidence in the physical exam does not have the time to come and verify findings at a patient's bedside with a curious learner.

This issue seeks to emphasize the physical examination in specific diseases. Almost by definition, if readers have made it this far in this issue, they desire to learn more about disease-specific physical findings. Acquiring mastery in the physical exam is a highly rewarding but challenging journey that only comes with many years spent in the company of patients. Knowledge of test characteristics—whether sensitivity and specificity or positive and negative likelihood ratios—requires dedicated study as well as humility about the fact that for some physical exam maneuvers, there are little data in the medical literature. The experienced practitioner of the physical exam recognizes that some findings may clinch a diagnosis—lid retraction and fine tremor in hyperthyroidism, for example—while others, such as the puddle sign in ascites, are practically useless and not worth subjecting patients to.

This issue attempts to build upon a foundation of curiosity on the part of the reader and upon the reader's desire to know more about disease-specific physical examination. The humble goal of this issue is to make the reader a better and more skilled clinician, and above and beyond that, to help patients receive the excellent care that they seek and deserve.

Paul Aronowitz, MD, MACP
Department of Medicine
University of California, Davis School of Medicine
4150 V Street, Suite 3100 PSSB
Sacramento, CA 95817, USA

E-mail address:
paronowitz@ucdavis.edu

Cancer

Kristen D. Kelley, MD, MAS[a],*, Paul Aronowitz, MD[b]

KEYWORDS

- Malignancy • Cancer • Physical examination • Lymphadenopathy
- Deep vein thrombosis • Sweet syndrome • Sign of Leser-Trélat • Cushing disease

KEY POINTS

- Unexplained lymphadenopathy is caused by cancer in approximately 1% of cases, and findings that increase likelihood of underlying malignancy include generalized lymphadenopathy, splenomegaly, and "B symptoms".
- There are numerous cutaneous findings associated with internal malignancy including acanthosis nigricans, the sign of Leser-Trlat, and Sweet syndrome.
- Up to 20% of first-time thrombotic events are malignancy related thus clinicians should perform a complete history and physical, basic lab testing, and age-appropriate cancer screenings, more extensive screening does not improve survival.

INTRODUCTION

Cancer is the second leading cause of death in the United States, following heart disease. In most cancers, early detection is one of the most important factors in determining prognosis. As clinicians it is therefore important to be aware of potential clues of underlying malignancy on the physical examination. Given the wide range of malignancies, and the heterogeneous nature of their presentations, this article is by no means exhaustive. Instead, this article discusses in depth some of the more frequently encountered physical examination findings that may suggest malignancy. Specifically, it covers lymphadenopathy, cutaneous findings related to various cancers, and malignancy-related thrombosis.

DISCUSSION
Lymphadenopathy

Lymphadenopathy, defined as lymph nodes that are abnormally large or have an abnormal consistency, is a relatively common finding with an estimated annual incidence of 0.6%.[1,2] There are a wide range of causes for lymphadenopathy, often taught by the mnemonic "MIAMI"—malignancy, infections, autoimmune, miscellaneous, and

a Division of General Internal Medicine, UC Davis Heath, 4150 V Street, Suite 2400, Sacramento, CA 95817, USA; b UC Davis Health, 4150 V Street, Suite 2400, Sacramento, CA 95817, USA
* Corresponding author.
E-mail address: kdkel@ucdavis.edu

Med Clin N Am 106 (2022) 411–422
https://doi.org/10.1016/j.mcna.2021.12.006
0025-7125/22/Published by Elsevier Inc.

iatrogenic (medications). In most cases, lymphadenopathy is relatively benign and self-limited. However, at times lymphadenopathy may herald more serious underlying disease. It is estimated that malignancy is the cause of unexplained lymphadenopathy in approximately 1.1% of cases in the general population, increasing significantly with age.[2] When lymphadenopathy is identified on examination, providers should complete a thorough evaluation to determine the presence of risk factors or "red flags" concerning for underlying malignancy.

There are several aspects of the physical examination, which can help guide the differential diagnosis, including whether the lymphadenopathy is localized or generalized, as well as which specific anatomic regions are involved. Generalized lymphadenopathy is defined as involving 2 or more noncontiguous groups of lymph nodes.[1] Generalized lymphadenopathy suggests a systemic cause, such as widespread infection, autoimmune process, or malignancy. A prospective study investigating outcomes of lymph node biopsy in patients with unexplained lymphadenopathy referred by primary care providers found that patients with generalized lymphadenopathy were more than 6 times as likely to have underlying malignancy compared with patients with localized lymphadenopathy.[3]

The location of affected lymph nodes is also a significant factor in considering how serious the lymphadenopathy may be. Historically, certain lymph nodes were associated with specific underlying disease, such as the "Virchow node," a left supraclavicular lymph node that was associated with metastatic gastric cancer.[4,5] However, it is more accurate to think of involved nodes based on anatomic regions of lymph drainage. The Virchow node is a site for lymph drainage through the thoracic duct and therefore may be involved in many other primary cancers that metastasize through this pathway.[4,6] It is probably most productive to consider the general anatomic regions involved when prioritizing the differential diagnosis. For example, head or neck lymphadenopathy (including the preauricular, submental, submandibular, anterior and posterior cervical, and supraclavicular regions) is most commonly caused by infections, such as upper respiratory infections or mononucleosis. However, other locations involving the supraclavicular and infraclavicular nodes are more concerning for malignancies such as lymphoma[1,3] (**Fig. 1** shows an example of large left supraclavicular lymph node in patient found to have acute lymphoblastic lymphoma).

The finding of splenomegaly in the presence of lymphadenopathy helps to narrow the differential diagnosis. Diseases known to cause both lymphadenopathy and splenomegaly include mononucleosis, lymphomas, and leukemias so that in patients with lymphadenopathy and splenomegaly in the absence of symptoms or signs of mononucleosis, malignancy should be a major concern.

The characteristics of enlarged lymph nodes—tender versus nontender or mobile versus fixed—are often described and used to prioritize the differential diagnosis. For example, tender lymphadenopathy is often due to inflammation and is usually associated with infection. However, these characteristics are nonspecific and cannot be fully relied upon because necrosis, bleeding, and rapid proliferation have all been associated with malignancies that may lead to tender lymph nodes.

In addition to physical examination findings, carefully considering patient demographic features and obtaining a thorough history can help narrow likely causes. One of the most important factors in weighing the likelihood of lymphadenopathy being due to underlying malignancy is patient age. A retrospective study investigating outcomes of lymph node biopsy found that in patients younger than 30 years only 21% of the biopsies revealed malignancy, compared with 60% of lymph node biopsies revealing malignancy in patients aged between 51 and 80 years.[7] Other

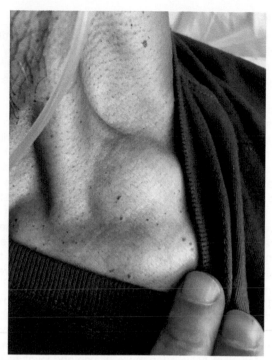

Fig. 1. Enlarged left supraclavicular lymph node in patient found to have acute lympho-blastic lymphoma. (*From* the collection of P. Aronowitz; with permission.)

important factors to consider are the presence of associated symptoms such as "B" symptoms, including fevers, night sweats, and unexplained weight loss, which raise concern for malignancy, particularly hematologic in origin. However, these historical points are also nonspecific and can be seen in some indolent infectious processes such as tuberculosis as well as fungal infections.

Key points

- Lymphadenopathy can represent a variety of underlying causes, often taught by the MIAMI mnemonic (malignancy, infection, autoimmune, miscellaneous, and iatrogenic)
- Unexplained lymphadenopathy is caused by malignancy in about 1% of cases, but increases in incidence with patient age
- Generalized lymphadenopathy suggests a systemic cause and also increases the likelihood of underlying malignancy
- Lymphadenopathy in the presence of splenomegaly suggests either mononucleosis or hematologic malignancy
- Qualitative characteristics of lymph nodes (tender or nontender, fixed or mobile) is nonspecific and generally is not reliable in prioritizing the differential diagnosis
- When considering malignancy as a potential cause of lymphadenopathy, one should carefully gather and consider the patient history for associated "B symptoms"—fatigue, fevers, night sweats, and unexplained weight loss.

Cutaneous Findings

Abnormal skin findings are a commonly encountered patient presenting concern, and some dermatologic findings may signify serious systemic disease, such as cancer. Although there are many documented cutaneous findings of internal malignancies, the focus here is on some of the more frequently encountered ones.

Acanthosis nigricans

Acanthosis nigricans (AN) is a relatively common cutaneous finding, and appears as hyperkeratotic, hyperpigmented plaques with a texture often described as "velvety." AN lesions most commonly occur on the flexure surfaces of the body such as the axillae and the posterior neck.[8] AN is usually a benign finding associated with obesity and insulin resistance. However, in some cases AN arises as a paraneoplastic syndrome associated with underlying malignancy. Malignant AN is most strongly associated with gastric carcinoma. A retrospective review of 277 cases of malignant AN found that 55% were associated with gastric carcinomas and another 18% with other intra-abdominal carcinomas.[9] Most commonly, malignant AN is detected at the same time that the diagnosis of cancer is made, but in about 18% of cases the finding of malignant AN can precede the malignancy diagnosis, in some cases preceding the diagnosis by several years.[10,11]

Given that AN may signal underlying malignancy, it is important to consider the features of AN that raise the most concern for malignancy. In general, the appearance and tempo of malignant AN is much more aggressive when compared with benign AN. Benign AN typically has an indolent progression, whereas malignant AN progresses rapidly.[12] Malignant AN is often more diffuse and involves sites not typically associated with benign AN such as the mucosal membranes, palms of the hands, or soles of the feet.[12,13] Another distinguishing factor is the age at which AN develops; benign AN most commonly develops in adolescence or young adulthood, whereas malignant AN more commonly develops in older patients. In summary, when considering the likelihood of AN being related to underlying malignancy, the following risk factors should be considered: older age of the patient, rapid progression, extensive involvement in atypical regions of the body (mucous membranes, palms and soles), and absence of obesity or insulin resistance.

Leser-Trélat sign

The sign of Leser-Trélat (SLT) is the sudden eruption of multiple, often pruritic, seborrheic keratoses, which is associated with internal malignancy.[14,15] Gastrointestinal adenocarcinomas, including gastric, liver, colorectal, and pancreatic, are the malignancies most commonly associated with SLT, although there are reports of a variety of other malignancies also being associated with SLT[16] (**Figs. 2** and **3** show a patient with SLT found to have adenocarcinoma of the colon). In almost 70% of cases, SLT is identified before a diagnosis of malignancy has been made and can also occur concurrently with malignant AN.[16] It is therefore important for providers to recognize SLT and initiate a prompt investigation for occult malignancy. Of note, a "pseudo-sign of Leser-Trélat" has also been described in which there is a similar rapid appearance and progression of seborrheic keratoses but is not associated with underlying cancer. Nonmalignant causes that can lead to this clinical finding include pregnancy, administration of chemotherapeutic agents, as well as various other benign conditions.

Sweet syndrome

Sweet syndrome, or acute febrile neutrophilic dermatosis, is characterized by the abrupt appearance of tender erythematous plaques or nodules, fever, and peripheral

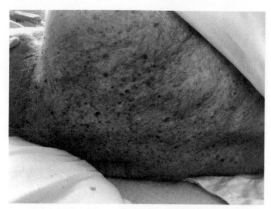

Fig. 2. Sign of Leser-Trélat in a patient with colonic adenocarcinoma. (*From* the collection of P. Aronowitz with permission.)

neutrophilia. When biopsied, pathology specimens demonstrate a neutrophil-predominant infiltrate in the dermis (**Figs. 4** and **5** demonstrate the cutaneous findings of Sweet syndrome). Sweet syndrome is associated with an underlying systemic process in approximately half the cases. Causes include infection (most commonly upper respiratory tract or gastrointestinal), inflammatory bowel disease, pregnancy, and medications. Approximately 20% of cases of Sweet syndrome are associated with an underlying malignancy.[17,18] Hematologic malignancies and myeloproliferative and myelodysplastic disorders are more commonly associated with Sweet syndrome in contrast to solid tumors, which are rarely an underlying cause.[18,19] The physical appearance of the lesions seen in Sweet syndrome does not help to distinguish Sweet syndrome related to malignancy from another cause. However, several studies have highlighted associated findings that increase the risk of malignancy-associated Sweet syndrome, which include thrombocytopenia, anemia, leukopenia, and the absence of arthralgias.[18,19] Without an identified cause of Sweet syndrome, age-appropriate cancer screening should be performed. The development of Sweet syndrome can precede a cancer diagnosis by several months leading some investigators to

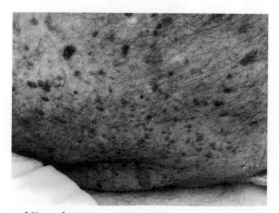

Fig. 3. Close up view of Sign of Leser-Trelat in a patient with colonic adenocarcinoma. (*From* the collection of P. Aronowitz; with permission.)

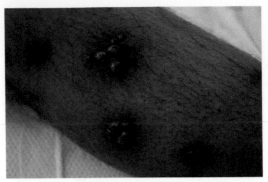

Fig. 4. Sweet syndrome cutaneous findings. (*From* the collection of P. Aronowitz; with permission.)

recommend that patients with Sweet syndrome without an obviously associated systemic condition be closely followed for at least 16 months to exclude underlying malignancy.[18]

Cushing syndrome
Cushing syndrome is the clinical manifestation of chronic exposure to excess glucocorticoids. There are a variety of causes of Cushing syndrome, with the most common being the exogenous administration of corticosteroids. Endogenous causes are

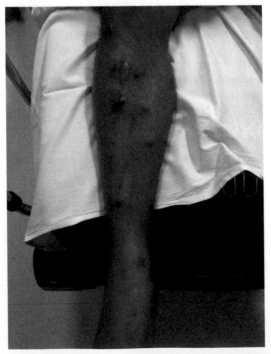

Fig. 5. Erythematous nodules on the leg in a patient with Sweet syndrome. (*From* the collection of P. Aronowitz; with permission.)

initially categorized in terms of dependence on adrenocorticotrophic hormone (ACTH). Corticotropin-releasing hormone (CRH) is released by the hypothalamus and stimulates the anterior pituitary to release ACTH, which then acts on the adrenal cortex to stimulate the release of glucocorticoids. Glucocorticoids then provide negative feedback on CRH and ACTH release, thus maintaining proper levels of glucocorticoids in the body.

In ACTH-dependent Cushing syndrome—accounting for 80% of endogenous cases—excess ACTH bypasses the feedback loop and leads to unregulated release of glucocorticoids from the adrenal gland.[20] The most common cause of ACTH-dependent Cushing syndrome is an ACTH-producing pituitary adenoma, also known as Cushing disease. Other causes of ACTH-dependent Cushing syndrome include ectopic ACTH production from tumors occurring beyond the pituitary gland, such as ACTH-producing neuroendocrine tumors. Ectopic ACTH production is less frequent, being the cause in approximately 5% to 10% of cases.[20]

In ACTH-independent Cushing syndrome, which makes up approximately 20% of cases of endogenous Cushing syndrome, the adrenal gland produces excess glucocorticoids independently of signals from the pituitary gland.[20] In these cases, the excess cortisol provides feedback to the hypothalamus and anterior pituitary to suppress ACTH, resulting in low ACTH levels when measured. The causes of ACTH-independent Cushing syndrome include benign glucocorticoid-producing adrenal adenomas and adrenal carcinomas.

There is a wide spectrum of clinical manifestations of Cushing syndrome ranging from subclinical to more severe manifestations such as early osteoporosis. Commonly reported symptoms in Cushing syndrome include fatigue, depression, decreased libido, weight gain, and menstrual changes in women. On physical examination, the most common findings are central obesity, "moon" facies, ecchymoses, dorsal fat pad, and facial plethora.[21] Many of these signs and symptoms are nonspecific to Cushing syndrome and are commonly seen in patients with other underlying processes. Studies have found that a collection of these findings, including easy bruising, facial plethora, proximal myopathy or proximal muscle weakness, and striae (especially if reddish-purple in color and great than 1 cm) have greater specificity for Cushing syndrome.[22,23] Because these findings have a higher specificity but low sensitivity for Cushing syndrome, their presence is highly suggestive of Cushing syndrome, but their absence does not rule out this disorder.

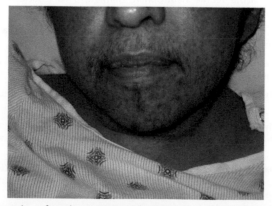

Fig. 6. Hirsutism seen in a female patient with virilization from adrenal carcinoma. (*From* the collection of P. Aronowitz; with permission.)

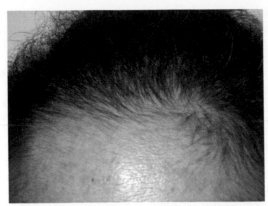

Fig. 7. Male pattern baldness seen in a female patient with virilization from adrenal carcinoma. (*From* the collection of P. Aronowitz; with permission.)

With regard to adrenal carcinomas, Cushing syndrome is the most commonly associated clinical syndrome—approximately 30% to 40% of patients with adrenal carcinoma will have Cushing syndrome.[24] Virilization, which presents in women as hirsutism, oligomenorrhea, male pattern baldness, and clitoromegaly, is seen along with other features of Cushing syndrome in 25% of patients with adrenal carcinoma[24] (**Figs. 6** and **7** show clinical signs of virilization in a patient found to have adrenal carcinoma). The presence of virilization in patients with Cushing syndrome is therefore an important clinical clue to the presence of adrenal carcinoma in patients presenting with Cushing syndrome.

Key points

- AN—usually associated with obesity and insulin resistance—can also signify the presence of an underlying malignancy, most commonly gastric carcinoma
- Malignancy-associated AN tends to be more extensive and has a faster onset than benign AN
- The SLT, an abrupt eruption of seborrheic keratoses, is associated with gastrointestinal malignancies but has also been reported to occur with other malignancies
- Sweet syndrome—acute febrile neutrophilic dermatosis—is associated with underlying malignancy in 20% of cases
- In patients presenting with Sweet syndrome, thrombocytopenia, anemia, leukopenia, and the absence of arthralgias suggest underlying malignancy
- Cushing syndrome is caused by excess exposure to glucocorticoids, and its most common cause is exogenous due to use of prescribed corticosteroids
- Endogenous causes of Cushing syndrome are categorized as ACTH dependent or ACTH independent
- Many of the physical examination findings in Cushing syndrome are nonspecific, but the most specific findings are easy bruising, facial plethora, proximal muscle weakness, and purple striae
- Physical examination findings of excessive virilization, including hirsutism, male pattern baldness, or clitoromegaly, should raise concern for underlying adrenal carcinoma as the cause of Cushing syndrome

Malignancy-Associated Thrombosis

The relationship between thrombosis and malignancy was first noted in the nineteenth century when Armand Trousseau described a relationship between the development of migratory thromboses and the presence of underlying visceral malignancy.[25] Remarkably, 2 years after first documenting this association, Trousseau discovered it on himself and subsequently died of gastric cancer.[26] The relationship between malignancy and thrombosis is now well recognized, and it is estimated that approximately 20% of cases of first-time acute venous thromboembolism are malignancy associated.[27,28] Discussion here focuses on lower extremity deep vein thrombosis (DVT) because this is a relatively commonly encountered condition, which is often first detected on physical examination.

Deep vein thrombosis

The classic triad of symptoms associated with lower extremity DVT includes asymmetric limb edema, pain, and erythema. However, the common clinical findings associated with DVT are not highly specific and are commonly seen in other disease processes. A large meta-analysis examined the diagnostic value of common clinical features of DVT. There were several features associated with a positive likelihood ratio (LR) for DVT being present. The presence of calf swelling was associated with a +LR of 1.45, meaning that this merely increased the probability of disease by less than 15%.[29] Other "classic" clinical findings associated with DVT had similarly unimpressive positive LRs, including calf tenderness (LR 1.27), calf warmth (LR 1.29), and difference in calf diameter (LR 1.8).[29] The "Homan sign," a physical examination maneuver in which the leg is extended at the knee and the foot is dorsiflexed and is considered positive when the maneuver elicits pain in the calf or popliteal region, had a nonsignificant LR relegating it to the list of useless physical examination tests no longer considered useful. In this study, the highest positive LR for deep venous thrombosis was the presence of malignant disease, which had an LR of 2.71. Given these rather underwhelming LRs for physical examination findings of DVT, there is not a single examination finding that can be relied upon in making the diagnosis of DVT; therefore a collection of findings along with patient risk factors for venous thrombosis must be relied upon to help inform the next steps in diagnostic testing.

One commonly used and validated clinical prediction tool is the "Wells criteria," which divides patients into low, moderate, and high probability of DVT categories, which then guide the next diagnostic steps. The "Wells criteria" takes into account risk factors, such as the presence of malignancy or recent surgery, as well as physical examination findings, such as calf swelling greater than 3 cm when compared with the opposite leg.[30] Patients in the high-probability category had an incidence of DVT of 75% compared with those in the low-probability group with an incidence of only 3%. Stratifying by pretest probability greatly informs decision making, leading to a recommendation that low- and moderate-probability patients undergo further risk stratification with D-dimer testing, whereas high-probability patients should undergo diagnostic imaging, most commonly ultrasonography.[31]

Following confirmation of a diagnosis of DVT, the next clinical question is to determine the cause, because this may impact the duration of treatment as well as patient prognosis. In many cases the cause of the DVT is clear on initial evaluation, such as in a patient with a hip fracture and surgical repair or in a patient with recent prolonged bed rest. However, in other cases the cause is not apparent after the initial history and evaluation; these cases are called "idiopathic DVTs." Approximately 5% to 10% of patients with idiopathic DVT, without evidence of malignancy on initial evaluation, will be diagnosed with malignancy within 1 year of initial DVT diagnosis[32,33]; this equates to approximately 4 to 6 times the risk of cancer as those in the general population. This observation raises the question of whether to perform extensive malignancy screening at the time of diagnosis of an idiopathic DVT. As extensive screening has not been shown to decrease patient mortality, currently it is not recommended.[34] A more limited evaluation for malignancy in patients with idiopathic DVT is recommended and includes a thorough history and physical examination, basic serum chemistries and complete blood cell count, and age-appropriate cancer screening.

Key points

- The association of malignancy and thrombosis has been long established, and it is estimated that up to 20% of first-time thrombotic events are malignancy related
- While physical examination findings in patients with lower extremity DVT may include asymmetric edema, erythema, and calf pain, these findings are not very sensitive or specific; clinicians should use these findings in connection with patient demographics and risk factors when considering DVT as a diagnosis
- Clinical decision models, such as the "Wells criteria," greatly improve the ability to assess the probability of DVT, and these models are useful in determining next diagnostic steps
- In the first year after idiopathic DVT diagnosis, there is a 5% to 10% incidence of detection of occult malignancy, which is 4 to 6 times greater than that of the general population
- Although extensive screening for malignancy increases the detection of occult cancers, it does not translate into improvement in survival
- Clinicians should perform limited screening for malignancy in patients diagnosed with idiopathic DVT, which includes a complete history and physical, basic blood tests, and age-appropriate cancer screening

---

SUMMARY

There are numerous physical examination findings that may suggest underlying malignancy, and identifying these findings can expedite appropriate workup and earlier diagnosis. This article focused on some of the more commonly encountered findings, including lymphadenopathy, cutaneous changes, and malignancy-associated thrombosis and explored what specific findings increase or decrease the likelihood of underlying malignancy.

CLINICS CARE POINTS

- Unexplained lymphadenopathy is caused by cancer in approximately 1% of cases, and findings that increase likelihood of underlying malignancy include generalized lymphadenopathy, splenomegaly, and associated "B symptoms"
- AN, although usually associated with benign causes such as obesity and insulin resistance, can at times be associated with internal malignancy
- Malignant AN is usually more rapid in onset and extensive in areas affected compared with benign AN
- The SLT, or the abrupt eruption of seborrheic keratoses, is also associated with internal malignancies, and can be seen in conjunction with AN
- Sweet syndrome, or acute febrile neutrophilic dermatosis, is associated with underlying malignancy in 20% of cases

- In Sweet syndrome, thrombocytopenia, anemia, leukopenia, and the absence of arthralgias suggest underlying malignancy

- Many findings in Cushing syndrome are nonspecific and seen in many disease processes; however, the most specific findings include easy bruising, facial plethora, proximal muscle weakness, and striae

- Additional findings of excessive virilization, such as hirsutism, male pattern baldness, or clitoromegaly, raise the concern for underlying adrenal carcinoma as the cause of Cushing syndrome

- First-time venous thromboembolic events are malignancy related in 20% of cases

- In the first year following diagnosis of an idiopathic DVT 5% to 10% of patients will be diagnosed with a malignancy

- After diagnosis of idiopathic DVT, clinicians should perform a thorough history and physical examination, obtain basic laboratory studies, and complete age-appropriate cancer screening; it is not recommended that more exhaustive screening for occult malignancy be undertaken because studies indicate that this does not impact mortality

DISCLOSURE

The authors have nothing to disclose.

REFERENCES

1. Gaddey HL, Riegel AM. Unexplained lymphadenopathy: evaluation and differential diagnosis. Am Fam Physician 2016;94(11):896–903.
2. Fijten GH, Blijham GH. Unexplained lymphadenopathy in family practice. An evaluation of the probability of malignant causes and the effectiveness of physicians' workup. J Fam Pract 1988;27(4):373–6.
3. Chau I, Kelleher MT, Cunningham D, et al. Rapid access multidisciplinary lymph node diagnostic clinic: analysis of 550 patients. Br J Cancer 2003;88(3):354–61.
4. Aghedo BO, Kasi A. Virchow node. Treasure Island (FL): StatPearls; 2021.
5. Karamanou M, Laios K, Tsoucalas G, et al. Charles-Emile Troisier (1844-1919) and the clinical description of signal node. J BUON 2014;19(4):1133–5.
6. Zdilla MJ, Aldawood AM, Plata A, et al. Troisier sign and Virchow node: the anatomy and pathology of pulmonary adenocarcinoma metastasis to a supraclavicular lymph node. Autops Case Rep 2019;9(1):e2018053.
7. Lee Y, Terry R, Lukes RJ. Lymph node biopsy for diagnosis: a statistical study. J Surg Oncol 1980;14(1):53–60.
8. Schwartz RA. Acanthosis nigricans. J Am Acad Dermatol 1994;31(1):1–19 [quiz: 20-12].
9. Rigel DS, Jacobs MI. Malignant acanthosis nigricans: a review. J Dermatol Surg Oncol 1980;6(11):923–7.
10. Thomas M, Radhakrishnan S, Sunny B, et al. Malignant acanthosis nigricans with occult primary. Indian J Dermatol Venereol Leprol 2002;68(6):371–3.
11. Krawczyk M, Mykala-Ciesla J, Kolodziej-Jaskula A. Acanthosis nigricans as a paraneoplastic syndrome. Case reports and review of literature. Pol Arch Med Wewn 2009;119(3):180–3.
12. Shah KR, Boland CR, Patel M, et al. Cutaneous manifestations of gastrointestinal disease: part I. J Am Acad Dermatol 2013;68(2):189–e181-121 [quiz: 210].
13. Stone SP, Buescher LS. Life-threatening paraneoplastic cutaneous syndromes. Clin Dermatol 2005;23(3):301–6.

14. Schwartz RA. Sign of Leser-Trelat. J Am Acad Dermatol 1996;35(1):88–95.
15. Holdiness MR. The sign of Leser-Trelat. Int J Dermatol 1986;25(9):564–72.
16. Husain Z, Ho JK, Hantash BM. Sign and pseudo-sign of Leser-Trelat: case reports and a review of the literature. J Drugs Dermatol 2013;12(5):e79–87.
17. Cohen PR, Kurzrock R. Sweet's syndrome and cancer. Clin Dermatol 1993;11(1): 149–57.
18. Marcoval J, Martin-Callizo C, Valenti-Medina F, et al. Sweet syndrome: long-term follow-up of 138 patients. Clin Exp Dermatol 2016;41(7):741–6.
19. Nelson CA, Noe MH, McMahon CM, et al. Sweet syndrome in patients with and without malignancy: a retrospective analysis of 83 patients from a tertiary academic referral center. J Am Acad Dermatol 2018;78(2):303–309 e304.
20. Lacroix A, Feelders RA, Stratakis CA, et al. Cushing's syndrome. Lancet 2015; 386(9996):913–27.
21. Nieman LK. Cushing's syndrome: update on signs, symptoms and biochemical screening. Eur J Endocrinol 2015;173(4):M33–8.
22. Nieman LK, Biller BM, Findling JW, et al. The diagnosis of Cushing's syndrome: an Endocrine Society Clinical Practice Guideline. J Clin Endocrinol Metab 2008;93(5):1526–40.
23. Ross EJ, Linch DC. Cushing's syndrome–killing disease: discriminatory value of signs and symptoms aiding early diagnosis. Lancet 1982;2(8299):646–9.
24. Ng L, Libertino JM. Adrenocortical carcinoma: diagnosis, evaluation and treatment. J Urol 2003;169(1):5–11.
25. Trousseau A, Bazire PV, Cormack JR. Lectures on clinical medicine. London (UK): R. Hardwicke; 1867.
26. Khorana AA. Malignancy, thrombosis and Trousseau: the case for an eponym. J Thromb Haemost 2003;1(12):2463–5.
27. Timp JF, Braekkan SK, Versteeg HH, et al. Epidemiology of cancer-associated venous thrombosis. Blood 2013;122(10):1712–23.
28. Heit JA, O'Fallon WM, Petterson TM, et al. Relative impact of risk factors for deep vein thrombosis and pulmonary embolism: a population-based study. Arch Intern Med 2002;162(11):1245–8.
29. Goodacre S, Sutton AJ, Sampson FC. Meta-analysis: The value of clinical assessment in the diagnosis of deep venous thrombosis. Ann Intern Med 2005;143(2): 129–39.
30. Wells PS, Anderson DR, Bormanis J, et al. Value of assessment of pretest probability of deep-vein thrombosis in clinical management. Lancet 1997;350(9094): 1795–8.
31. Wells PS, Anderson DR, Rodger M, et al. Evaluation of D-dimer in the diagnosis of suspected deep-vein thrombosis. N Engl J Med 2003;349(13):1227–35.
32. van Es N, Le Gal G, Otten HM, et al. Screening for occult cancer in patients with unprovoked venous thromboembolism: a systematic review and meta-analysis of individual patient data. Ann Intern Med 2017;167(6):410–7.
33. Delluc A, Antic D, Lecumberri R, et al. Occult cancer screening in patients with venous thromboembolism: guidance from the SSC of the ISTH. J Thromb Haemost 2017;15(10):2076–9.
34. Robin P, Otten HM, Delluc A, et al. Effect of occult cancer screening on mortality in patients with unprovoked venous thromboembolism. Thromb Res 2018; 171:92–6.

Chronic Obstructive Pulmonary Disease and the Physical Examination

Reeni Ann Abraham, MD*, Stephanie Kaye Brinker, MD

KEYWORDS

- Chronic obstructive pulmonary disease • Physical examination • History taking
- Diagnosis • Comorbidities

KEY POINTS

- Use key clinical risk factors and symptoms in the history to inform a hypothesis-driven physical examination.
- A history of chronic obstructive pulmonary disease (COPD) should prompt a physical examination that looks for common signs of frequently associated comorbidities.
- Various auscultatory and percussive physical examination maneuvers can help predict the likelihood of COPD.
- Certain physical examination signs are present in severe COPD and should initiate key management strategies.

INTRODUCTION

Chronic obstructive pulmonary disease (COPD) is a common and preventable medical condition. The diagnosis of COPD requires a history of ongoing respiratory symptoms and evidence of airflow limitation, usually measured by spirometry.[1] Growing in prevalence, COPD is the third leading cause of death in the United States and the fourth leading cause of death globally.[2] By 2060, it is predicted that 5.4 million deaths will occur each year secondary to COPD and related comorbid conditions alone. Currently, developing and under-resourced countries account for the overwhelming majority of the deaths from COPD.[1]

Although the cardinal respiratory symptoms of COPD are common in the primary care setting, COPD remains underdiagnosed, with various studies reporting only 9.4% to 30% of patients with COPD having been diagnosed.[3,4] The early detection and diagnosis of COPD can decrease COPD exacerbations and improve the quality of life of patients through interventions including smoking cessation, vaccination

Division of General Internal Medicine, UT Southwestern Medical Center, 5323 Harry Hines Boulevard, Mail Code 9030, Dallas, TX 75390, USA
* Corresponding author.
E-mail address: reeni.abraham@utsouthwestern.edu

Med Clin N Am 106 (2022) 423–435
https://doi.org/10.1016/j.mcna.2022.02.001
0025-7125/22/© 2022 Elsevier Inc. All rights reserved.

medical.theclinics.com

against influenza, and initiation of medications including bronchodilators and inhaled steroids.[5–7] History-taking and physical examination maneuvers are the most cost-effective way for health care providers to screen patients for the need of further work-up and to monitor severity of COPD.[8]

DEFINITION

COPD is diagnosed when a patient has both persistent respiratory symptoms of either dyspnea, cough or sputum production and confirmed airflow limitation with forced expiratory volume in 1 second (FEV_1)/forced vital capacity (FVC) less than 0.70 caused by airway and/or alveolar abnormalities (**Fig. 1**).[2] The Global Initiative for Chronic Obstructive Lung Disease (GOLD) program specifically has removed the terms emphysema and chronic bronchitis previously highlighted when defining COPD.[1]

When the GOLD program was initiated in 1998, COPD was solely classified according to the FEV_1, which was thought to directly correlate with disease progression. Subsequently, FEV_1 has been found to be a poor indicator of symptom burden.[9,10] The development and use of validated symptom questionnaires, translated and available in multiple languages, have transformed the GOLD staging system and incorporated patient symptoms along with spirometry cut-offs to target COPD management strategies and thereby impact short-term and long-term clinical outcomes.[1]

RISK FACTORS

Many structural and downstream social and biological factors are associated with respiratory development and affect access to or the presence of irritants that cause the lung and systemic inflammation found in patients with COPD (**Fig. 2**).[1] The presence of any of these risk factors should prompt further investigation of accompanying symptoms and additional risk factors on history-taking and subsequently a hypothesis-driven physical examination to improve detection of COPD.

Smoking and Other Environmental Factors

Smoking is the most common risk factor for developing COPD, with studies reporting at least 50% of cases of COPD mortality are attributed to smoking, irrespective of

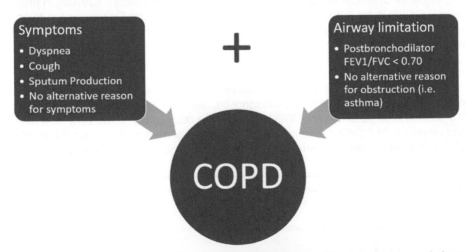

Fig. 1. Diagnosis of COPD requires presence of certain persistent symptoms and documented airway limitation, with no alternative etiologies.

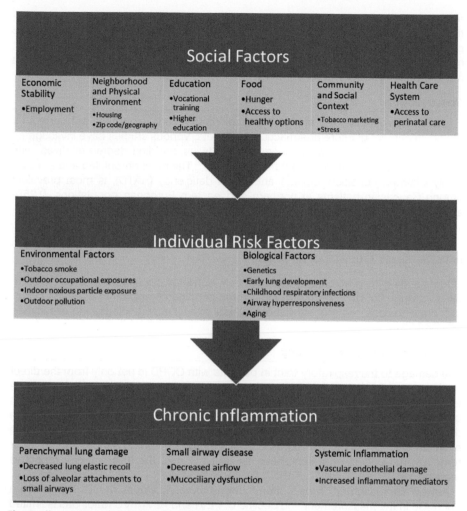

Fig. 2. Illustration of the interplay of various social factors, using the Kaiser Family Foundation's Social Determinants of Health model, individual risk factors, and the resulting inflammatory response found in patients with COPD.[20]

gender.[11] Occupational exposure to dust, gas, and fumes such as in coal and hard-rock mining may also account for another 15% to 20% of cases. In other populations, such as women and those in developing countries, common environmental factors with strong evidence of association with the development of COPD include outdoor air pollution and biomass smoke from cooking over an open fire.[12]

Perinatal and Early Childhood Factors

Mechanisms are not completely understood, but much research has focused on effects of perinatal and early childhood events on disease. Specifically, in chronic lung disease, maternal obesity, intrauterine growth restriction (IUGR), and childhood obesity are well-studied risk factors resulting in bronchial hypercontractility, tissue degeneration, and lung remodeling.[13] Airway hyper-responsiveness is a significant risk factor for COPD, with a documented approximately 15% attributable risk, and patients with asthma were found to have a 12-fold risk of developing COPD compared to patients without asthma.[1] Lesser-studied risk factors include home overcrowding, high pollution exposure, presence of infant respiratory infection, and belonging to a manual working social class.[14,15]

Genetic Factors

The evolving understanding of the genetic role in COPD development is important for the advancement of future pharmaceutical targets. Various studies have investigated the relationship of COPD risk among siblings, twins, and first-degree relatives, with findings consistent with significant heritable risk.[16] The most chronicled and a recessively inherited condition, alpha-1 antitrypsin deficiency (AATD), is most prevalent among Caucasian patients in northern and eastern European populations, 0.25% and 0.08% respectively, although there are also rare incidences among African American patients.[1]

PATHOBIOLOGY AND PATHOPHYSIOLOGY

Understanding the physiologic processes by which known risk factors cause the pathologic changes of COPD can help explain the condition's relation to common symptom presentations, the progression of physical examination findings, and associated comorbidities.

Chronic Inflammation of the Lung

The damage to the respiratory tract in patients with COPD is not only from the direct noxious stimuli irritation but the inflammatory response that is initiated and then amplified. Mechanisms of action include oxidative stress and excess levels of both proteases, which cause connective tissue degradation, and inflammatory cells in the peripheral airways, lung parenchyma, and pulmonary vessels. This cascade eventually leads to airway fibrosis and emphysematous changes. Even after removing the underlying irritant, such as tobacco use, the inflammatory response remains.[1]

Airway narrowing and fibrosis often found in the early stages of COPD produce a decrease in the measurement and decline of FEV_1 and FEV_1/FVC ratio. Gas is limited in its ability to escape during expiration, causing hyperinflation, an early sign of the disease that can be identified on physical examination, which worsens with exertion. This decrease in functional capacity may lead to a natural and subconscious decline in physical activity and falsely reduce reporting of symptoms.[17] As the severity of the disease worsens, gas exchange abnormalities increase.

Another key symptom of COPD is persistent phlegm production from increased inflammatory mediators. Although these changes do not always result in an airflow limitation and are not present in all patients, these symptoms may be bothersome to patients, and increased during exacerbations.[18]

Chronic Inflammation and Consequences

Another late development in the COPD disease course is concomitant progressively worsening inflammatory vascular changes, such as endothelial cell dysfunction. It is thought that hypoxic vasoconstriction leads to intimal hyperplasia and smooth muscle hypertrophy and hyperplasia. In emphysematous changes, a decrease of the pulmonary capillary bed leads to increases in pulmonary hypertension, which is independently associated with COPD exacerbations and cor pulmonale.[1]

The inflammatory response of COPD may cause and worsen medical conditions such as coronary artery disease, heart failure, osteoporosis, and metabolic syndrome. The ongoing hypoxemia, systemic inflammation, and functional decline may also result in neurocognitive impairment and depression and/or anxiety.[19] Late sequelae of the inflammatory cascade may also lead to profound muscle wasting and cachexia.[1]

HYPOTHESIS-DRIVEN APPROACH TO THE HISTORY AND PHYSICAL EXAMINATION

COPD should be in the differential diagnosis in any patient presenting with dyspnea, chronic cough or sputum production, or recurrent lower respiratory infections. Utilizing the known risk factors and common symptom presentations, a hypothesis-driven approach to history-taking can inform which physical examination maneuvers should be performed to increase the post-test probability of a diagnosis and inform appropriate diagnostic work-up (**Box 1**).[21]

Although smoking is by far the most common risk factor for the development of COPD, screening every smoker with spirometry for COPD without clinical signs and symptoms is not practical and is not recommended by the US Preventative Services Task Force.[22] Multiple studies have shown that at this time there is no single history or examination finding pathognomonic for COPD.[23,24] However, when the history and physical examination are taken in concert, they can raise the likelihood of the COPD diagnosis, increasing the pretest probability of confirmatory spirometry.

Dyspnea is among the most common presenting symptoms in primary care clinics and emergency rooms. The differential diagnosis for dyspnea is often broad and includes cardiovascular disease, other lung diseases, and COPD, particularly in older patients who smoke tobacco.

Box 1
The medical history for a patient with known or suspected chronic obstructive pulmonary disease

- Identify exposure to risk factors: smoking, occupational, and environmental exposures
- Elicit a history of asthma, allergy, sinusitis or nasal polyps, childhood respiratory tract infections, or other chronic respiratory diseases
- Explore family history of COPD or other chronic respiratory disease
- Consider pattern of symptom development: more likely to be adult onset; patients may report more frequent upper respiratory infections, and progressive dyspnea
- Question history of exacerbations or previous hospitalizations for respiratory disorders: episodes that may not have been recognized as COPD exacerbations
- Look for presence of comorbidities: cardiovascular disease, metabolic syndrome, osteoporosis, skeletal muscle dysfunction, depression and anxiety, and malignancies, as these influence morbidity and mortality and contribute to restriction of activity
- Assess disease impact on patient's life: limitation of activity, economic impact, and effect on mental health and sexual activity
- Identify the patient's social and family support
- Explore possibilities for reducing risk factors, especially smoking cessation

Adapted from the Global strategy for the Diagnosis, Management, and Prevention of Chronic Obstructive Pulmonary Disease, 2021 Report[1].

Taking a Chronic Obstructive Pulmonary Disease Hypothesis-Driven History

The medical history should focus on identifying the patient's risk factors for COPD, assessing disease impact on the patient's function, looking for disease-modifiable factors and identifying comorbidities that impact morbidity and mortality in COPD. Metanalyses have shown COPD is associated with significantly higher comorbidities than other diseases.[25]

When looking at what findings from the patient history are most predictive of COPD, analyses have shown that only the complaints of dyspnea, wheezing, prior reported history of treatment for wheezing or cough, self-reported COPD, age of at least 45 years, female sex, symptoms provoked by allergens, and smoking either currently or greater than 40 pack-year history have independent diagnostic value.[26] The strongest diagnostic indicators were symptoms provoked by allergens (odds ratio = 4.5), wheezing (odds ratio = 4.4), greater than 40 pack-years (+ likelihood ratio = 11.6) and self-reported COPD (+ likelihood ratio = 4.4).[26]

Performing a Chronic Obstructive Pulmonary Disease Hypothesis-Driven Examination

There are numerous observational, palpatory, and auscultatory physical examination findings that have been described in COPD patients in the literature with variable predictive value. Although most have a relatively low sensitivity and specificity for COPD, there are a few key maneuvers that can significantly increase post-test probability of the diagnosis of COPD. Overall, by the time physical signs of airflow limitation are present on examination, significant impairment of lung function has occurred.[9]

Among physical examination findings observed in COPD patients, hyper-resonance to percussion has been described as a strong predictor of COPD. This test is performed by percussing the lung fields in the anterior and posterior chest and is characterized by an increased hollow sound. Oshaug and colleagues[27] found that this examination maneuver has a sensitivity of 20.8 and a specificity of 97.8, with a likelihood ratio (LR) of 9.6.

Another individual physical examination finding that independently increases the likelihood of COPD when found are early inspiratory crackle (+ LR 14.6), although this is based on 2 small studies only.[28,29]

Diminished breath sound intensity (BSI) is frequently described in COPD patients. Clinician report of diminished breath sounds alone is described as a predictor of COPD.[27] When utilizing a scoring system by which the clinician auscultates 6 locations over the patient's chest and assigns intensity scores to each area, the diminished breath sounds become a strong predictor of COPD. Using this system, the examiner auscultates bilaterally over the upper anterior chest, in the midaxilla, and at the posterior bases, and assigns an intensity score of 0 for absent sounds, 1 for barely audible sounds, 2 for faint but heard sounds, 3 for normal sounds, and 4 for louder than normal sounds. The scores are added, and a total BSI score of no more than 9 has an LR of 10.2 for chronic airflow obstruction, but a score of at least 16 decreases the probability (LR = 0.1).[30]

Combining the Patient's History with Other Physical Examination Findings Also Improves Diagnostic Accuracy

When the patient history is combined with physical examination findings, the diagnostic accuracy is increased. For example, when the breath sound intensity score is used in combination with the history, the diagnostic accuracy is increased. A proposed combined model by Badgett and colleagues asked:

- Has the patient smoked for more than 70 pack-years?
- Is there a previous diagnosis of emphysema or chronic bronchitis?
- Are breath sounds diminished?

Answering yes to 2 of these questions has positive LR of 33.5 for the diagnosis of COPD.[31]

Several physical examination findings related to hyperinflation of the lungs become highly significant with combined history. Patients with COPD have been noted to have many physical examination findings specifically related to hyperinflation of the lungs, including loss of the expected cardiac dullness and a dullness to percussion over the left sternal boarder in the fifth intercostal space. Absent cardiac dullness alone has a sensitivity of 16% and specificity of 99% for moderate COPD. However, in a patient with a smoking history or self-reported COPD, cardiac dullness has a positive LR of 16. Conversely, the negative LR is only 0.8 for the diagnosis of COPD, meaning that an absence of normal cardiac dullness in a smoker is helpful in the prediction of COPD, but present cardiac dullness is not helpful to rule out the diagnosis.[31]

Another assessment of hyperinflation is laryngeal height measured from the top of the thyroid cartilage to the suprasternal notch. Hyperinflation of the lungs shortens the laryngeal height by displacing the clavicles and sternum upwards, and diaphragmatic contraction pulls the trachea downward in COPD patients. A maximal tracheal height of no more than 4 cm has a positive LR of 5.21 for COPD, but when this finding is combined with a screening tool, the Lung Function Questionnaire (queries age, smoking history, frequency of productive cough, chest sounds, and dyspnea on exertion), the positive LR of COPD increases to 29.06.[32]

Differential Diagnosis

A patient with cardiovascular risk factors presenting with progressive dyspnea and productive cough would likely prompt consideration of heart failure and pneumonia in addition to COPD, among other etiologies. Findings from the patient history and physical examination signs can be organized into illness scripts to differentiate between common presentations of dyspnea. These history and physical examination findings and their likelihood ratios can be taken together to raise and lower the pretest probability of COPD versus other common diagnoses for dyspnea in patients with comorbid conditions like aging and smoking (**Table 1**).

EVALUATION OF THE CHRONIC OBSTRUCTIVE PULMONARY DISEASE PATIENT WITH PROGRESSIVELY WORSENING SYMPTOMS

The evaluation of patients with advanced COPD should be focused on eliciting a history of anorexia, worsening dyspnea, cough, fatigue, and syncope. Dyspnea, cough, and fatigue are the hallmarks of advanced COPD and are sometimes called the respiratory cluster.[41]

Weight loss and loss of muscle mass are common physical examination findings in advanced COPD that have prognostic importance. When admitted to the hospital for COPD exacerbations, patients found to have significant muscle loss have increased length of stay, increased health care costs, and higher in-hospital mortality.[42] The findings of muscle and fat loss are associated with increased mortality in COPD.[43]

Patients with COPD should be also screened for depression and anxiety during the history. Comorbidity of COPD and depression leads to increased risk of exacerbations and poorer health status. Depression is more prevalent in people with COPD compared with those without COPD, and even mild symptoms of depression more than double the risk of emergency room visits regardless of COPD disease severity.[41]

Table 1
Illness scripts for common differential diagnoses of dyspnea

	Chronic Obstructive Pulmonary Disease	Pneumonia	Congestive Heart Failure
History	Smoking	Subjective Fever	Orthopnea
	Wheezing or coughing	Cough	Paroxysmal nocturnal dyspnea
	Reported COPD	After upper respiratory tract infection	Bendopnea
	Symptoms worsened by allergens	Structural lung disease	Lower extremity edema
	Demographic: age > 45, female sex	Older age	
Physical Exam	Diminished breath sounds (+ LR 33.5 with history)[31]	Asymmetric chest expansion (+ LR 44.1, -LR 1.0)[33]	Jugular venous distention $\geq$ 8 cm (+ LR 9.7, -LR 0.3)[34,35]
	Absent cardiac dullness (+ LR 16, - LR 0.8 with history)[31]	Egophony (+ LR 6.8, -LR 0.9)[33,36]	Jugular venous distention $\geq$12 cm (+LR 10.4, -LR 0.1)[34,35,37]
	Hyper-resonance to percussion (+LR 9.6)[27]	Dullness to percussion (over lung fields) (+ LR 5.7, -LR 0.9)[33,36]	Abdominojugular reflux (+ LR 8.0, -LR 0.3)[38]
	Laryngeal height < 4 cm (+ LR 29.6 with history)[31]	Bronchophony (+ LR 3.3, -LR 0.9)[36]	Displaced apical impulse (+ LR 10.3, -LR 0.7)[39,40]
	Early inspiratory crackles (+ LR 14.6)[28,29]	Decreased breath sounds (+LR 2.5, -LR 0.7)[36]	
		Crackles (+LR 3.2, -LR 0.7)[33,36]	

The history and examination should also look for the development of pulmonary hypertension and cor pulmonale in patients with worsening symptoms. Patients with right-sided heart failure may report increased dyspnea on exertion, exertional chest pain, syncope, dizziness, cough, and hemoptysis. These patients may present with a wide variety of physical examination findings including lower extremity, right ventricular heave, and signs of tricuspid regurgitation.[44] However, the physical examination is unreliable for determining the presence of pulmonary hypertension (**Box 2**).[45]

Determining prognosis for patients with COPD has greatly evolved over the years, and recent studies have shown that specific concomitant comorbidities significantly increase mortality risk, including certain cancers, pulmonary fibrosis, atrial fibrillation/flutter, coronary artery disease, congestive heart failure, gastric/duodenal ulcers, liver cirrhosis, diabetes with neuropathy, and anxiety. The risk index calculator, the COPD-specific comorbidity test (COTE), is used in conjunction with other prognostic disease risk indices, such as the body mass index, FEV_1, dyspnea, and exercise capacity (BODE) to calculate the mortality risk for these patients.[46] These comorbidities are the major drivers of increased mortality, higher medical costs, and worsened health outcomes for patients with COPD.[19]

Given severe symptom burden and functional decline seen with advanced COPD, experts advocate for early palliative care interventions integrated with both COPD

Box 2
History and physical examination signs of severe disease in chronic obstructive pulmonary disease

History

Anorexia[42]

Syncope: due to rapid increase in intrathoracic pressure during prolonged paroxysms of cough[44,45]

Depression and anxiety: exacerbated by breathlessness, fear of disease, social isolation, loss of function[47]

Breathlessness[41]

Cough[41]

Fatigue[41]

Physical Examination Signs

Weight loss[42]

Muscle atrophy[42]

Depressed mood[47]

Signs of Cor Pulmonale

Lower extremity edema,

Displaced PMI

Right ventricular heave

Tricuspid regurgitation[45]

Evidence of hypoxia: cyanosis, clubbing[45]

---

services to treat the fatigue and dyspnea with pulmonary rehabilitation to improve functional status, quality of life, and breathlessness.[41] Evidence shows improvement in quality of life without cost increase with early integration of palliative care, a practice endorsed by the American Thoracic Society.[48]

SUMMARY

Performing a hypothesis-driven examination in patients with possible COPD can increase the recognition and diagnosis of this life-threatening and costly medical condition. While a history of cough, dyspnea and sputum production should always prompt consideration of COPD, eliciting high-yield risk factors during the patient history and using known likelihood ratios for specific physical examination maneuvers can adjust a patient's pretest probability of having COPD and inform appropriate diagnostic work-up. Recognition of comorbid conditions and examination findings suggestive of end-stage COPD can mitigate the decreased quality of life and mortality of multi-morbidity and instigate earlier palliative measures.

CLINICS CARE POINTS

Pearls

Key history findings for COPD include: symptoms provoked by allergens, wheezing, greater than 40 pack-years history of smoking, and self-reported COPD.[23]

Key physical examination findings for COPD include diminished breath sounds, absent cardiac dullness at the fifth intercostal space/left lower sternal border,[49] hyper-resonance to percussion,[27] and early inspiratory crackles.[28,29]

When history and physical examination findings are combined, diagnostic accuracy is improved.

Pitfalls

COPD is an under-diagnosed but life-threatening disease. No single physical examination finding is pathognomonic[23,24,50]

COPD is frequently found comorbid with other chronic diseases. Comorbidities have implications on the morbidity and mortality of COPD.[51]

End-stage COPD patients are frequently referred too late to palliative care. Recognition of history and physical examination findings suggestive of end-stage COPD should prompt referral for palliative interventions.[48,52]

DISCLOSURES

Nothing to disclose by all authors.

REFERENCES

1. Global Initiative for Chronic Obstructive Lung Disease. Global strategy for the diagnosis, management, and prevention of chronic obstructive pulmonary disease. 2021. Available at: https://goldcopd.org/2021-gold-reports/. Accessed August 15, 2021.
2. Duffy SP, Criner GJ. Chronic obstructive pulmonary disease: evaluation and management. Med Clin North Am 2019;103(3):453–61.
3. Bednarek M, Maciejewski J, Wozniak M, et al. Prevalence, severity and underdiagnosis of COPD in the primary care setting. Thorax 2008;63(5):402–7.
4. Quach A, Giovannelli J, Chérot-Kornobis N, et al. Prevalence and underdiagnosis of airway obstruction among middle-aged adults in northern France: the ELISABET study 2011-2013. Respir Med 2015;109(12):1553–61.
5. Anthonisen NR, Connett JE, Murray RP. Smoking and lung function of lung health study participants after 11 years. Am J Respir Crit Care Med 2002;166(5):675–9.
6. Bekkat-Berkani R, Wilkinson T, Buchy P, et al. Seasonal influenza vaccination in patients with COPD: a systematic literature review. BMC Pulm Med 2017; 17(1):79.
7. Calverley PM, Anderson JA, Celli B, et al. Salmeterol and fluticasone propionate and survival in chronic obstructive pulmonary disease. N Engl J Med 2007; 356(8):775–89.
8. Sarkar M, Bhardwaz R, Madabhavi I, et al. Physical signs in patients with chronic obstructive pulmonary disease. Lung India 2019;36(1):38–47.
9. Çolak Y, Nordestgaard BG, Vestbo J, et al. Prognostic significance of chronic respiratory symptoms in individuals with normal spirometry. Eur Respir J 2019;54(3).
10. Jackson H, Hubbard R. Detecting chronic obstructive pulmonary disease using peak flow rate: cross sectional survey. BMJ 2003;327(7416):653–4.
11. Ezzati M, Lopez AD. Estimates of global mortality attributable to smoking in 2000. Lancet 2003;362(9387):847–52.
12. Eisner MD, Anthonisen N, Coultas D, et al. An official American Thoracic Society public policy statement: novel risk factors and the global burden of chronic obstructive pulmonary disease. Am J Respir Crit Care Med 2010;182(5):693–718.

13. Kuiper-Makris C, Selle J, Nüsken E, et al. Perinatal nutritional and metabolic pathways: early origins of chronic lung diseases. Front Med (Lausanne) 2021;8: 667315.
14. Gauderman WJ, Avol E, Gilliland F, et al. The effect of air pollution on lung development from 10 to 18 years of age. New Engl J Med 2004;351(11):1057–67.
15. Allinson JP, Hardy R, Donaldson GC, et al. Combined impact of smoking and early-life exposures on adult lung function trajectories. Am J Respir Crit Care Med 2017;196(8):1021–30.
16. Silverman EK. Genetics of COPD. Annu Rev Physiol 2020;82:413–31.
17. McDonough JE, Yuan R, Suzuki M, et al. Small-airway obstruction and emphysema in chronic obstructive pulmonary disease. New Engl J Med 2011; 365(17):1567–75.
18. Burgel PR, Nadel JA. Epidermal growth factor receptor-mediated innate immune responses and their roles in airway diseases. Eur Respir J 2008;32(4):1068–81.
19. Putcha N, Drummond MB, Wise RA, et al. Comorbidities and chronic obstructive pulmonary disease: prevalence, influence on outcomes, and management. Semin Respir Crit Care Med 2015;36(4):575–91.
20. Artiga SH, Hinton E. Beyond health care: the role of social determinants in promoting health and health equity. 2018. Available at: https://www.kff.org/racial-equity-and-health-policy/issue-brief/beyond-health-care-the-role-of-social-determinants-in-promoting-health-and-health-equity/. Accessed September 12, 2021.
21. Garibaldi BT, Olson APJ. The hypothesis-driven physical examination. Med Clin North America 2018;102(3):433–42.
22. Screening for chronic obstructive pulmonary disease using spirometry: U.S. Preventive Services Task Force recommendation statement. Ann Intern Med 2008; 148(7):529–34.
23. Broekhuizen BD, Sachs AP, Hoes AW, et al. Diagnostic management of chronic obstructive pulmonary disease. Neth J Med 2012;70(1):6–11.
24. Holleman DR Jr, Simel DL. Does the clinical examination predict airflow limitation? JAMA 1995;273(4):313–9.
25. Yin HL, Yin SQ, Lin QY, et al. Prevalence of comorbidities in chronic obstructive pulmonary disease patients: a meta-analysis. Medicine (Baltimore) 2017;96(19): e6836.
26. Broekhuizen BD, Sachs AP, Oostvogels R, et al. The diagnostic value of history and physical examination for COPD in suspected or known cases: a systematic review. Fam Pract 2009;26(4):260–8.
27. Oshaug K, Halvorsen PA, Melbye H. Should chest examination be reinstated in the early diagnosis of chronic obstructive pulmonary disease? Int J Chron Obstruct Pulmon Dis 2013;8:369–77.
28. Nath AR, Capel LH. Inspiratory crackles and mechanical events of breathing. Thorax 1974;29(6):695–8.
29. Bettencourt PE, Del Bono EA, Spiegelman D, et al. Clinical utility of chest auscultation in common pulmonary diseases. Am J Respir Crit Care Med 1994;150(5 Pt 1):1291–7.
30. Pardee NE, Martin CJ, Morgan EH. A test of the practical value of estimating breath sound intensity. Breath sounds related to measured ventilatory function. Chest 1976;70(03):341–4.
31. Badgett RG, Tanaka DJ, Hunt DK, et al. Can moderate chronic obstructive pulmonary disease be diagnosed by historical and physical findings alone? Am J Med 1993;94(2):188–96.

32. Casado V, Navarro SM, Alvarez AE, et al. Laryngeal measurements and diagnostic tools for diagnosis of chronic obstructive pulmonary disease. Ann Fam Med 2015;13(1):49–52.

33. Diehr P, Wood RW, Bushyhead J, et al. Prediction of pneumonia in outpatients with acute cough–a statistical approach. J Chronic Dis 1984;37(3):215–25.

34. Davison R, Cannon R. Estimation of central venous pressure by examination of jugular veins. Am Heart J 1974;87(3):279–82.

35. Sankoff J, Zidulka A. Non-invasive method for the rapid assessment of central venous pressure: description and validation by a single examiner. West J Emerg Med 2008;9(4):201–5.

36. Heckerling PS, Tape TG, Wigton RS, et al. Clinical prediction rule for pulmonary infiltrates. Ann Intern Med 1990;113(9):664–70.

37. Ducas J, Magder S, McGregor M. Validity of the hepatojugular reflux as a clinical test for congestive heart failure. Am J Cardiol 1983;52(10):1299–303.

38. Butman SM, Ewy GA, Standen JR, et al. Bedside cardiovascular examination in patients with severe chronic heart failure: importance of rest or inducible jugular venous distension. J Am Coll Cardiol 1993;22(4):968–74.

39. Ewy GA. The abdominojugular test: technique and hemodynamic correlates. Ann Intern Med 1988;109(6):456–60.

40. Fahey T, Jeyaseelan S, McCowan C, et al. Diagnosis of left ventricular systolic dysfunction (LVSD): development and validation of a clinical prediction rule in primary care. Fam Pract 2007;24(6):628–35.

41. Maddocks M, Lovell N, Booth S, et al. Palliative care and management of troublesome symptoms for people with chronic obstructive pulmonary disease. Lancet 2017;390(10098):988–1002.

42. Attaway AH, Welch N, Hatipoğlu U, et al. Muscle loss contributes to higher morbidity and mortality in COPD: an analysis of national trends. Respirology 2021;26(1):62–71.

43. Hanania NA, Müllerova H, Locantore NW, et al. Determinants of depression in the ECLIPSE chronic obstructive pulmonary disease cohort. Am J Respir Crit Care Med 2011;183(5):604–11.

44. Crawford MHSA, Aras M, Sanchez J. Quick dx & rx: cardiology. New York: McGraw-Hill Education; 2019.

45. Colman R, Whittingham H, Tomlinson G, et al. Utility of the physical examination in detecting pulmonary hypertension. A mixed methods study. PLoS One 2014; 9(10):e108499.

46. Divo M, Cote C, de Torres JP, et al. Comorbidities and risk of mortality in patients with chronic obstructive pulmonary disease. Am J Respir Crit Care Med 2012; 186(2):155–61.

47. Blakemore A, Dickens C, Chew-Graham CA, et al. Depression predicts emergency care use in people with chronic obstructive pulmonary disease: a large cohort study in primary care. Int J Chron Obstruct Pulmon Dis 2019;14:1343–53.

48. Lanken PN, Terry PB, Delisser HM, et al. An official American Thoracic Society clinical policy statement: palliative care for patients with respiratory diseases and critical illnesses. Am J Respir Crit Care Med 2008;177(8):912–27.

49. Badgett RG, Tanaka DJ, Hunt DK, et al. The clinical evaluation for diagnosing obstructive airways disease in high-risk patients. Chest 1994;106(5):1427–31.

50. Alsaeedi A, Sin DD, McAlister FA. The effects of inhaled corticosteroids in chronic obstructive pulmonary disease: a systematic review of randomized placebo-controlled trials. Am J Med 2002;113(1):59–65.

51. Maselli DJ, Bhatt SP, Anzueto A, et al. Clinical epidemiology of COPD: insights from 10 years of the COPDGene study. Chest 2019;156(2):228–38.
52. Farquhar MC, Prevost AT, McCrone P, et al. The clinical and cost effectiveness of a breathlessness intervention service for patients with advanced non-malignant disease and their informal carers: mixed findings of a mixed method randomised controlled trial. Trials 2016;17:185.

Cirrhosis

Rachel Wilson, DO[a], Donna M. Williams, MD[b],*

KEYWORDS

- Cirrhosis • Liver • Ascites • Jaundice • Encephalopathy • Edema
- Physical examination • Spider nevi

KEY POINTS

- Cirrhosis is a chronic condition that develops over many years and results in a myriad of physical examination findings.
- Many signs and symptoms associated with liver disease are nonspecific, but some findings, such as dilated abdominal veins, ascites, encephalopathy, abnormal hair distribution, and gynecomastia, are more specific and suggest underlying cirrhosis.
- Early identification of physical findings that suggest cirrhosis can guide the clinician to order testing aimed at determining the underlying cause of cirrhosis, provide lifestyle counseling to avoid progression of disease, and suggest appropriate treatment and screening recommendations.

INTRODUCTION

Cirrhosis is a chronic condition resulting from inflammation and fibrosis of the liver. Fibrosis leads to distortion of the normal architecture of the liver and formation of nodules.[1] This process happens slowly, typically over decades, and leads to changes in blood flow through the liver as well as disruption of normal hepatocellular function. The gold standard for diagnosing cirrhosis is liver biopsy. Previously, cirrhosis was thought to be irreversible; however, recent evidence supports the idea that advanced fibrosis and even cirrhosis can be reversible with treatment of the underlying cause.[2] Although mortality rates for cirrhosis and hepatocellular carcinoma from all causes had been increasing in the United States between 2007 and 2016, mortality rates significantly declined for hepatitis C–related cirrhosis starting in 2014 due to the availability of direct-acting antiviral therapy.[3]

Author contributions: All authors contributed to drafting and critical revision of the article.
Conflict of Interest Disclosure: D.M. Williams's spouse is a co-founder and co-owner of Certus Critical Care, Inc, a medical device company. They currently have no devices on the market. R. Wilson reports no conflict of interest.

[a] University of Wisconsin School of Medicine and Public Health, 2828 Marshall Court, Suite 100, Madison, WI 53705, USA; [b] Section on General Internal Medicine, Wake Forest School of Medicine, Medical Center Boulevard, Winston Salem, NC 27157, USA
* Corresponding author.
E-mail address: dowillia@wakehealth.edu

The most common causes of cirrhosis in the United States include alcoholic liver disease, viral hepatitis, and nonalcoholic fatty liver disease.[4] Other, less common causes include autoimmune hepatitis, primary biliary cholangitis, cardiac cirrhosis, hemochromatosis, Wilson disease, cryptogenic cirrhosis, and others. Regardless of the cause, the complications of cirrhosis are similar and include bleeding due to decreased clotting factors; sequelae of increased portal pressure including esophageal varices and ascites; thrombocytopenia due to splenic sequestration; and decreased production of thrombopoietin, hepatic encephalopathy, infection, and renal failure.

In the clinical setting, patients are often categorized as having compensated or decompensated cirrhosis based on symptoms. Patients with compensated disease may present without any symptoms, whereas decompensated cirrhosis is often marked by variceal bleeding, ascites, or hepatic encephalopathy. The rate of transition from compensated to decompensated cirrhosis has been noted to be 4% to 10% per year, with an associated significant increase in mortality.[5]

Patients with cirrhosis may have a myriad of physical examination findings that reflect the severity of the underlying liver disease.[1] Although many signs and symptoms related to cirrhosis are nonspecific, such as abdominal pain, nausea, and malaise, some findings are more specific and point to complications of liver disease. In the next section, the authors discuss common physical examination maneuvers and findings that are relevant in cirrhosis. Where possible, likelihood ratios (LR) will be used to measure the utility of the examination maneuver or physical finding in the diagnosis of cirrhosis. Likelihood ratios are diagnostic weights that help clinicians interpret the physical examination findings of individual patients. Positive likelihood ratios greater than 1 increase the probability that the patient has the disease in question, where higher numbers denote increased significance. Negative likelihood ratios less than 1 decrease the probability that the patient has the disease in question, where lower numbers denote increased significance and thereby help to rule out a particular disease being looked for.[6]

HEPATOMEGALY AND THE LIVER EXAMINATION

When considering the diagnosis of cirrhosis, the abdominal examination, specifically the liver examination, plays an important role. There are 2 main methods for evaluating liver size at the midclavicular line (MCL). One method uses percussion alone, whereas another uses percussion on the superior aspect of the liver border and palpation or percussion on the inferior aspect. Although livers vary in size and shape based on gender and body habitus, it is expected that liver size less than 12 to 13 cm at the MCL rules out hepatomegaly.[7] Although occasionally used in clinical practice, newer studies suggest that the "scratch method" is subpar to palpation and percussion and should not be used when evaluating the liver.[8]

If the liver is palpable, this does not necessarily indicate enlarged liver size but does increase the likelihood of hepatomegaly. Conversely, the probability of hepatomegaly is reduced if a liver is nonpalpable.[7] When evaluating patients with chronic liver disease for the presence of cirrhosis, the positive likelihood ratio is 2.3 if hepatomegaly is present, with a negative likelihood ratio of 0.6 if hepatomegaly is not observed.[9]

Multiple other physical examination maneuvers investigating the liver can be performed to aid in the diagnosis of cirrhosis. The examination with the highest likelihood ratio to indicate cirrhosis is a firm liver edge on palpation, which has a positive likelihood ratio of 3.3.[9] Other findings, such as a palpable liver in the epigastrium, can also be helpful in the diagnosis of cirrhosis. As the liver changes, the left lobe atrophies when compared with the right lobe, and the liver is more easily palpated as the tissue becomes more firm. Patients with cirrhosis also have alterations in their body habitus, leading to wasting of abdominal musculature, which allows for easier palpation.[10] If the liver is palpable in the epigastrium, the likelihood ratio for cirrhosis is 2.7. Conversely, if it is not palpated in the epigastrium, the chance of cirrhosis decreases, as the negative likelihood ratio is 0.3.[9]

SPLENOMEGALY

Splenomegaly can be found in patients with hematological disorders, infectious diseases, or hepatic diseases. In a small subset of patients (3%–12%), splenomegaly can be a normal variant.[11] Examination of the spleen is challenging, however can be quite useful when splenomegaly is identified. Splenomegaly is defined as a spleen that is 13 cm or greater in cephalocaudal diameter as identified by ultrasound.[11] Most of the available data support the use of percussion and palpation for the detection of splenomegaly on physical examination, although confirmation with ultrasound is usually required.

There are 3 main percussion techniques used to examine the spleen: percussion via the Nixon method, percussion via the Castell method, and percussion of the Traube space.[11] Although all 3 of these techniques have been validated by ultrasound to confirm validity in detecting splenomegaly, the Nixon method and percussion of Traube space are slightly more reliable. In the evaluation of splenomegaly, the Castell method has a positive LR of 1.7, the Nixon method has a positive LR of 2.0, and Traube space dullness has a positive LR of 2.1.[12]

Evaluation of the spleen via palpation may have higher accuracy than percussion. There are 3 main techniques used to evaluate spleen size via palpation: two-handed palpation with the patient in the right lateral decubitus position, one-handed palpation with the patient supine, and the hooking maneuver of Middleton with patient supine. The supine one-handed palpation has the most data to support this method.[11] If the spleen is palpable by any technique, the positive LR of having splenomegaly is 8.5.[12] By performing both percussion and palpation together, the detection of splenomegaly is more likely.

In addition to the finding of splenomegaly, other examination findings aid in identification of underlying pathology. If a patient has both splenomegaly and lymphadenopathy, underlying hepatic disease is less likely (LR of 0.04).[12] In patients with cirrhosis, the associated portal hypertension leads to increased portal venous pressure gradient with resultant splenomegaly.[13] The probability of cirrhosis in patients with underlying liver disease and splenomegaly has a positive LR of 2.5 and negative LR of 0.8.[9]

JAUNDICE

Jaundice refers to yellow discoloration of the skin, which occurs due to pigment buildup, most commonly bilirubin. Although bilirubin can stain all tissue, jaundice is typically most prominent in the face, mucosal membranes, trunk, and conjunctiva (**Fig. 1**). It is typically not visible unless serum bilirubin levels are at least 3 mg/dL or higher. When considering causes of jaundice other than hepatic dysfunction, it is important to note whether the discoloration is evenly distributed throughout the conjunctiva, as other causes of yellow discoloration (such as carotenemia) are not uniform across the sclera and skin.[14] Jaundice in the setting of chronic liver disease has a positive likelihood ratio of 3.8 supporting the diagnosis of cirrhosis, whereas the negative likelihood is 0.8.[9]

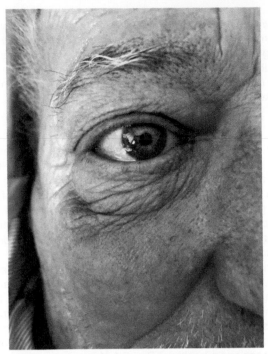

Fig. 1. Scleral icterus and jaundice of the skin. (Image courtesy of Paul Aronowitz, MD, Sacramento, CA.)

ASCITES

If a patient reports abdominal distention or increasing girth, it is important to identify the underlying cause. It may be due to feces, gas within the bowel, pregnancy, abdominal mass, fat, or fluid. Pathologic fluid accumulation in the abdomen is known as ascites. Over time, cirrhosis can progress to the development of portal hypertension, salt and fluid retention, and subsequent accumulation of ascites. A diagnostic paracentesis with calculation of the serum to ascites albumin gradient aids in identifying the underlying pathology that led to ascites. Eighty-four percent of cases of ascites are due to cirrhosis.[15] Other causes include pancreatitis, nephrotic syndrome, cardiac ascites, peritoneal carcinomatosis, infections (especially peritoneal tuberculosis), massive hepatic metastasis, and other rare causes.

History and physical examination are helpful in determining the presence of ascites. Typically, at least 1500 mL of fluid must be present in the abdomen in order to be detected by physical examination. Therefore, a clinician's inability to detect fluid on examination does not reliably exclude the diagnosis.[16] The gold standard for diagnosis of ascites is ultrasound, as it can detect volumes as small as 100 mL.[15]

The 4 main examination findings that suggest underlying ascites include fluid wave, bulging flanks, flank dullness, and shifting dullness. If present, the fluid wave has the highest positive likelihood ratio of 5.0. Shifting dullness follows this with a positive likelihood ratio of 2.3. Although these maneuvers are specific to the abdomen, it is important to examine the patient as a whole. If edema is detected on examination in addition to abdominal distention, the likelihood ratio of having underlying ascites is 3.8.[12]

When assessing for ascites, the lack of certain examination findings can be just as helpful as the presence of others. The absence of edema in the setting of abdominal distension decreases the probability of ascites with a negative likelihood ratio of 0.2. Flank tympany (or absence of flank fullness) has a negative LR of 0.3. The absence of bulging flanks and/or shifting dullness both decrease the probability of ascites with a negative likelihood ratio of 0.4.[12]

Diagnosing ascites and determining the underlying pathology is critical for patient care. Examination findings help guide the clinician to the diagnosis of ascites, increase clinical suspicion for spontaneous bacterial peritonitis (SBP), and suggest the need for timely paracentesis in order to guide patient care. SBP is a hallmark complication of ascites in which the fluid becomes infected; this is relatively common and can be deadly if left untreated or if treatment is delayed.

ENCEPHALOPATHY

In the setting of cirrhosis, vascular shunting and decreased liver mass can result in the accumulation of gut-derived neurotoxins in the body.[1] This build-up leads to encephalopathy, which can progress to coma if left untreated. Other conditions also present with encephalopathy without the presence of underlying cirrhosis, including hypertensive emergency, uremia, toxic ingestions, and others.

The physical examination is crucial for making the diagnosis of encephalopathy. Families may notice changes in patients' personalities, decreased mental sharpness, or disruption of the sleep-wake cycle, which often prompts presentation to a health care provider. On examination, the patient's mental status can vary from somnolent to agitated. If the patient is alert enough to participate in an examination, outstretched arms with wrist extension can produce asterixis, which is also known as a "flap." Clinicians pair these findings to make the clinical diagnosis of encephalopathy.

If encephalopathy is present in patients with chronic liver disease, the likelihood ratio for underlying cirrhosis is 8.8.[9] If hepatic encephalopathy is present, it is critical to look for the underlying trigger of this decompensation. Infections, electrolyte derangements, infections such as SBP, and gastrointestinal bleeding are common inciting events for hepatic encephalopathy.[1] Of note, although serum ammonia levels are found to be elevated in hepatic encephalopathy, the levels do not correspond to the severity of the underlying disease and cannot be monitored to assess for disease progression or improvement.

DILATED ABDOMINAL VEINS

Abdominal wall veins become dilated when venous obstruction is present and collateral blood flow subsequently develops. Most commonly, this is due to portal hypertension, but it can be due to other causes such as thrombosis, extrinsic compression of the superior or inferior vena cava, and other less common causes. By examining the direction of the blood flow within the dilated vessels, a clinician can distinguish between potential etiologies.[14] The examiner must evaluate the blood flow both in cranial to umbilicus and caudal to umbilicus directions.[13] If portal hypertension is the underlying cause, the blood will flow away from the umbilicus in cranial and caudal directions.

Cirrhosis is one of the primary causes of portal hypertension with subsequent abdominal vein dilation. This dilation can result in a venous rosette around the umbilicus, termed caput medusae. If a caput medusae is present in patients with underlying liver disease, the positive likelihood ratio for cirrhosis is 9.5.[9] Although not a common finding, dilated abdominal wall veins have the highest likelihood ratio of all physical examination findings, indicating the presence of cirrhosis (**Fig. 2**).

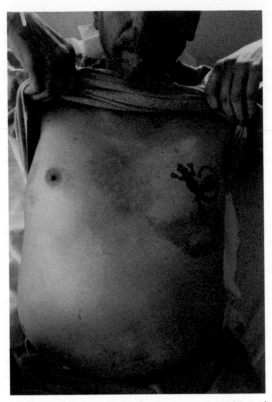

Fig. 2. Dilated abdominal wall veins, bulging flanks, gynecomastia, and ecchymosis in a patient with cirrhosis. (Image courtesy of Paul Aronowitz, MD, Sacramento, CA.)

SPIDER NEVI

Spider nevi are known by a variety of names: arterial spiders, vascular spiders, spider telangiectasias, or spider angiomas (**Fig. 3**). They are named for their appearance, as they have a central erythematous area with multiple "spider legs" made up of arterialized capillaries. They blanch on compression with quick return of blood into the central arteriole following release. Spider nevi are primarily located on the face and neck; less commonly they are found on the shoulders, chest, back, and arms, but they are rarely found below the umbilicus.[17] They are seen in 10% to 15% of healthy children and adults and can be present in other conditions such as pregnancy and rheumatoid arthritis and can be associated with medications such as oral contraceptives.

The presence of multiple spider nevi typically indicates cirrhosis.[18] It is thought that elevated circulating sex hormone activity in the setting of cirrhosis contributes to their development. When diagnosing cirrhosis in a patient with chronic liver disease, the presence of spider nevi has a positive likelihood ratio of 4.2 and negative likelihood ratio of 0.5.[9] In patients with chronic liver disease, spider nevi are more commonly seen in alcoholic patients than nonalcoholic patients. However, the presence of spider nevi correlates with a higher risk of death in patients with cirrhosis from any cause.[19]

PALMAR ERYTHEMA

Palmar erythema refers to symmetric erythema located on the thenar and hypothenar eminences. Similar to spider nevi, palmar erythema is associated with liver disease,

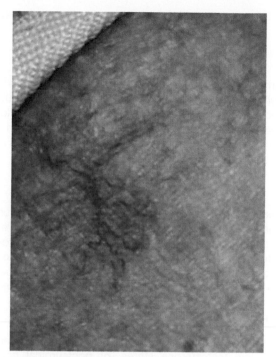

Fig. 3. Spider nevus. (Image courtesy of Paul Aronowitz, MD,Sacramento, CA.)

pregnancy, other less common pathologies, and even can even be hereditary. Although the exact mechanism is unclear, palmar erythema in cirrhotic patients is thought to be related to abnormal serum estradiol to testosterone level and changes in vasculature.[20] If found in patients with underlying liver disease, palmar erythema has a positive likelihood ratio of 3.7, which suggests cirrhosis.[9]

PERIPHERAL EDEMA

Bilateral peripheral pitting edema can result from abnormalities in cardiac, renal, or hepatic function or rarely due to bilateral venous thromboembolic disease. When evaluating edema, the clinical presentation is critical in the determination of the underlying cause. In patients with cirrhosis, low albumin states, especially with serum albumin less than 3.0 g/dL, as well as poor venous return due to pressure on the inferior vena cava from the ascites both contribute to the development of edema. For patients with chronic liver disease, the presence of peripheral edema has a positive likelihood ratio of 3.0, suggesting cirrhosis.[9] As noted when evaluating for ascites, the absence of peripheral edema decreases the probability of ascites with a negative likelihood ratio of 0.2.[12]

ABNORMAL HAIR DISTRIBUTION

Patients with cirrhosis often have reduction in body, axillary, and pubic hair.[21] Hair loss is thought to be related to hormone imbalances involving estrogen and testosterone. Abnormal hair distribution is most common in patients with cirrhosis, and it is not typically found in simple liver disease.[22] If abnormal hair distribution is found in patients with chronic liver disease, the positive likelihood ratio of having underlying cirrhosis is 8.8.[9]

GYNECOMASTIA

Because of abnormal hormone levels, male patients with cirrhosis can develop gynecomastia. Specifically, gynecomastia is glandular breast tissue that is palpable, 2 to 3 cm in size, and located under the areola. On physical examination, it is important to distinguish between true gynecomastia and fatty tissue deposition. Often, true glandular tissue is tender, whereas adipose tissue is not.[23] If seen in liver disease, gynecomastia has a positive likelihood ratio of 7.0 to diagnose cirrhosis.[9]

BODY HABITUS

Up to 40% of patients with cirrhosis develop muscle wasting. As the underlying pathology progresses, the incidence of wasting increases.[24] Multiple factors contribute to the development of muscle wasting including poor nutrition, altered protein metabolism, the liver's inability to successfully regulate protein production, and modified absorption of nutrients in the bowels.[1] As a result, cirrhotics can live in a catabolic state and are often cachectic on examination with significant, diffuse muscular atrophy.

TESTICULAR ATROPHY

Testicular atrophy may be present in patients with a variety of underlying conditions, including cirrhosis, low testosterone states, or postsurgical complications after inguinal surgery repair. If other physical examination findings suggest cirrhosis, this diagnosis should be considered. Approximately 40% to 50% of men with cirrhosis will develop testicular atrophy and gynecomastia.[25] These changes occur in the setting of hormone imbalances related to the underlying cirrhosis.

TERRY NAILS

Terry nails are found in patients with cirrhosis, congestive heart failure, diabetes, or increased age.[26] Bilaterally, the nails seem white at the base with extension toward the distal nail. The white discoloration can conceal the underlying lunula and progress to cover the entire nail bed except the distal 1 to 2 mm. These findings are most prominently found in the thumb and index finger.[27]

FETOR HEPATICUS

Dimethyl sulfide in the breath causes a characteristic odor in cirrhotic patients known as fetor hepaticus.[28] The smell is distinct and described as an odor similar to a mixture of garlic and rotten eggs. Although not a common finding, its presence is due to shunting in the setting of cirrhosis rather than actual liver failure or encephalopathy.[9]

SUMMARY

The physical examination can be helpful in identifying patients who have underlying cirrhosis, especially if historical features such as alcohol or drug use, known diagnosis of viral hepatitis, or obesity are present. Many patients with cirrhosis have compensated disease, which can be present chronically without the need for hospitalization. Decompensated cirrhosis, including the presence of ascites, acute gastrointestinal bleeding often from esophageal varices, and hepatic encephalopathy, often drives patients to seek emergency care and frequently requires hospitalization. Early identification of physical findings that suggest cirrhosis can guide the clinician to order testing aimed at determining the underlying cause of cirrhosis, provide lifestyle counseling to avoid progression of disease, and suggest appropriate treatment and screening recommendations.

CLINICS CARE POINTS

- When evaluating patients with chronic liver disease for the presence of cirrhosis, the liver examination with the highest likelihood ratio to indicate cirrhosis is a firm liver edge on palpation, which has a positive likelihood ratio of 3.3.[9]

- Jaundice in the setting of chronic liver disease has a positive likelihood ratio of 3.8, supporting the diagnosis of cirrhosis whereas the negative likelihood is 0.8.[9]

- When assessing a patient for the presence of ascites, the fluid wave has the highest positive likelihood ratio of 5.0. Shifting dullness follows this with a positive likelihood ratio of 2.3.

- If encephalopathy is present in patients with chronic liver disease, the likelihood ratio for underlying cirrhosis is 8.8.[9]

- Although not a common finding, dilated abdominal veins have the highest likelihood ratio of all physical examination findings of cirrhosis with a positive LR of 9.5.[9]

- When diagnosing cirrhosis in a patient with chronic liver disease, the presence of spider nevi has a positive likelihood ratio of 4.2 and negative likelihood ratio of 0.5.[9]

- If abnormal hair distribution is found in patients with chronic liver disease, the positive likelihood ratio of having underlying cirrhosis is 8.8.[9]

REFERENCES

1. Bacon BR. Cirrhosis and Its Complications. In: Jameson L, Fauci AS, Kasper DL, et al, editors. Harrison's Principles of Internal Medicine, 20e. McGraw Hill; 2018. Available at: https://accessmedicine.mhmedical.com/content.aspx?bookid=2129&sectionid=192283819. October 11, 2021.
2. Sohrabpour AA, Mohamadnejad M, Malekzadeh R. Review article: the reversibility of cirrhosis. Aliment Pharmacol Ther 2012;36:824–32.
3. Kim D, Li AA, Perumpail BJ, et al. Changing trends in etiology-based and ethnicity-based annual mortality rates of cirrhosis and hepatocellular carcinoma in the United States. Hepatology 2019;69:1064–74.
4. Smith A, Baumgartner K, Bositis C. Cirrhosis: diagnosis and management. Am Fam Physician 2019;100:759–70.
5. Asrani SK, Devarbhavi H, Eaton J, et al. Burden of liver diseases in the world. J Hepatol 2019;70(1):151–71.
6. McGee SR. Diagnostic Accuracy of Physical Exam Findings. In: Evidence-based physical diagnosis. 4th edition. Philadelphia (PA): Elsevier; 2018. p. 5–16.
7. Naylor CD. The rational clinical examination. Physical examination of the liver. JAMA 1994;271(23):1859–65.
8. Simel DL, Rennie D, Keitz SA. The rational clinical examination: evidence-based clinical diagnosis. New York: McGraw-Hill; 2009.
9. McGee SR. Jaundice. In: Evidence-based physical diagnosis. 4th edition. Philadelphia (PA): Elsevier; 2018. p. 59–68.
10. McCormick PA, Nolan N. Palpable epigastric liver as a physical sign of cirrhosis: a prospective study. Eur J Gastroenterol Hepatol 2004;16(12):1331–4.

11. Grover SA, Barkun AN, Sackett DL. The rational clinical examination. Does this patient have splenomegaly? JAMA 1993;270(18):2218–21 [published correction appears in JAMA. 2011 Apr 13;305(14):1414].

12. McGee SR. Palpation and Percussion of the Abdomen. In: Evidence-based physical diagnosis. 4th edition. Philadelphia (PA): Elsevier; 2018. p. 433–44.

13. Udell JA, Wang CS, Tinmouth J, et al. Does this patient with liver disease have cirrhosis? JAMA 2012;307(8):832–42.

14. The Abdomen, Perineum, Anus, and Rectosigmoid. In: Suneja M, Szot JF, LeBlond RF, Brown DD, editors. DeGowin's Diagnostic Examinatin, 11e. McGraw Hill; 2020. Available at: https://accessmedicine.mhmedical.com/content.aspx?bookid=2927&secionid=247756769. July 15, 2021.

15. Corey KE, Friedman LS. Abdominal Swelling and Ascites. In: Jameson J, Fauci AS, Kasper DL, et al, editors. Harrison's Principles of Internal Medicine, 20e. McGraw Hill; 2018. Available at: https://accessmedicine-mhmedical-com.ezproxy.library.wisc.edu/content.aspx?bookid=2129&sectionid=192013028. Se ptember 23, 2021.

16. Williams JW Jr, Simel DL. The rational clinical examination. Does this patient have ascites? How to divine fluid in the abdomen. JAMA 1992;267(19):2645–8.

17. The Skin and Nails. In: Suneja M, Szot JF, LeBlond RF, Brown DD, editors. DeGowin's Diagnostic Examination, 11e. McGraw Hill; 2020. Available at: https://accessmedicine.mhmedical.com/content.aspx?bookid=2927&sectionid=2477-53822. July 15, 2021.

18. Khasnis A, Gokula RM. Spider nevus. J Postgrad Med 2002;48(4):307–9.

19. Reuben A. Along came a spider. Hepatology 2002;35(3):735–6.

20. Serrao R, Zirwas M, English JC. Palmar erythema. Am J Clin Dermatol 2007;8(6):347–56.

21. Niederau C, Lange S, Frühauf M, et al. Cutaneous signs of liver disease: value for prognosis of severe fibrosis and cirrhosis. Liver Int 2008;28(5):659–66.

22. Schenker S, Balint J, Schiff L. Differential diagnosis of jaundice: report of a prospective study of 61 proved cases. Am J Dig Dis 1962;7:449–63.

23. Fitzgerald PA. Gynecomastia. In: Papadakis MA, McPhee SJ, Rabow MW, editors. Current Medical Diagnosis & Treatment 2021. McGraw Hill; 2020. Available at: https://accessmedicine.mhmedical.com/content.aspx?bookid=2957&sectionid=249377353. July 21, 2021.

24. Kalafateli M, Konstantakis C, Thomopoulos K, et al. Impact of muscle wasting on survival in patients with liver cirrhosis. World J Gastroenterol 2015;21(24):7357–61.

25. Green GR. Mechanism of hypogonadism in cirrhotic males. Gut 1977;18(10):843–53.

26. Holzberg M, Walker HK. Terry's nails: revised definition and new correlations. Lancet 1984;1(8382):896–9.

27. Terry R. White nails in hepatic cirrhosis. Lancet 1954;266(6815):757–9.

28. Tangerman A, Meuwese-Arends MT, Jansen JB. Cause and composition of foetor hepaticus. Lancet 1994;343(8895):483.

Congestive Heart Failure

Jennifer Chen, MD[a],*, Paul Aronowitz, MD, MACP[b]

KEYWORDS

- Congestive heart failure • Valsalva • Jugular venous pressure

KEY POINTS

- In patients with known or suspected heart failure, physical examination findings provide important prognostic information and can guide both diagnosis and management.
- The initial examination in a patient with shortness of breath should be approached in a "head-to-toe" manner with additional special maneuvers such as the measurement of jugular venous pressure (JVP), valsalva maneuver, and hepatojugular reflux performed as needed if there is suspicion for heart failure.
- After establishing a pretest probability based on prevalence and patient history, the examiner may then use clinical examination findings in conjunction with their positive and negative likelihood ratios to determine the posttest probability of heart failure as a diagnosis.

 Video content accompanies this article at http://www.medical.theclinics.com.

INTRODUCTION

Heart disease is the leading cause of death in the United States and has been estimated to affect 26 million people worldwide with greater than 1 million hospitalizations annually in both the United States and Europe.[1] It is estimated that approximately 6 million adults over the age of 20 in the United States are currently living with heart failure.[2] This prevalence has been increasing since the 1970s, largely attributed to an aging population, therapeutic advances in the treatment of heart failure which have improved the prognosis of the disease, as well as a rise in associated conditions which include hypertension and coronary artery disease.[3]

Many modern-day physicians rely heavily on imaging and laboratory testing to guide their diagnosis and medical management of heart failure rather than on physical examination skills. This has led some clinicians to question the utility of the physical examination in today's practice, at least as it applies to congestive heart failure.[4,5] Despite this skepticism, the medical literature indicates that examination findings continue to provide important prognostic information and can guide management in patients with

[a] Department of Internal Medicine, University of California, Davis, 4860 Y Street Suite 0100, Sacramento, CA 95817, USA; [b] Department of Internal Medicine, University of California, Davis, 4150 V Street Suite 3100 PSSB, Sacramento, CA 95817, USA
* Corresponding author.
E-mail address: jecchen@ucdavis.edu

Med Clin N Am 106 (2022) 447–458
https://doi.org/10.1016/j.mcna.2021.12.002
0025-7125/22/Published by Elsevier Inc.

medical.theclinics.com

congestive heart failure independently of laboratory tests and imaging.[4,6] The physical examination can aid in determining the need for hospitalization versus outpatient management and is a cost-effective method of guiding additional testing and interpretation of test results.[7]

One example of the value of the physical examination is in the setting of patients who present with shortness of breath, a common issue prompting patients to seek medical advice. The differential diagnosis is very broad for this chief complaint and includes cardiac, pulmonary, renal, and hepatic causes, among others. Congestive heart failure is frequently a major consideration in the adult patient, and the constellation of physical examination findings present in this disorder provides information on the posttest probability of the diagnosis and can guide targeted diagnostic workup and treatment regardless of the availability of echocardiography or other laboratory testing. Though echocardiogram and brain-type natriuretic peptide (BNP) are commonly used in the evaluation of suspected heart failure, the initial physical examination and subsequent focused, serial examination aids in the initial diagnosis and further monitoring and adjustment of medications and treatment. In fact, despite medical advances, laboratory and technology-driven guidance in the treatment of heart failure can sometimes prove dubious as a randomized clinical trial showed that BNP-guided therapy did not improve time to first hospitalization or decrease cardiovascular mortality in patients with reduced ejection fraction (EF).[8]

This article will focus on the approach to the physical examination in patients with suspected or known heart failure. Of note, there are 2 types of heart failure categories based on left ventricular ejection fraction (LVEF): heart failure with reduced ejection fraction (HFrEF) which is diagnosed based on an LVEF of less than or equal to 40% and heart failure with preserved ejection fraction (HFpEF) which is characterized by an LVEF of greater than or equal to 50%.[9] Both types of heart failure present with similar symptoms and physical examination findings, but determining the type of heart failure has important implications in medical management. Further discussion of the 2 types of heart failure other than as they apply to the physical examination is outside the scope of this review.

SYMPTOMS OF HEART FAILURE

Patients with heart failure may present with a variety of symptoms. Common complaints include:

1. Dyspnea or dyspnea on exertion (DOE)
2. Peripheral edema
3. Orthopnea: This is positional dyspnea that occurs when the patient is in the supine position and is often relieved with sitting or standing.[10] Orthopnea in the setting of heart failure is usually associated with an elevated pulmonary capillary wedge pressure (PCWP) and can assist with evaluating whether left ventricular filling pressures are elevated.[6]
4. Paroxysmal nocturnal dyspnea (PND): This is a sensation of shortness of breath during sleep that can awaken a patient and often resolves once the patient is upright.
5. Bendopnea: This is a recently described symptom whereby patients have shortness of breath with bending forward. It is associated with elevated filling pressures[11] and can be elicited by having the patient bend forward and touch their feet while sitting in a chair. Bendopnea is present if shortness of breath occurs within 30 seconds of bending.[6]

Nonspecific symptoms include fatigue, nausea, cough, wheezing (cardiac asthma), anorexia, and weight gain.

Given the prevalence of heart failure in the United States, it should be always be considered in the differential diagnosis for adult patients presenting with any of the above symptoms. In this article, we will discuss the general approach to the physical examination in the patient presenting with symptoms commonly associated with heart failure, with a particular focus on special maneuvers that may be performed if there is a strong suspicion for congestive heart failure.

APPROACH TO THE PHYSICAL EXAM

As with most disease-based physical examination, the physical examination for patients presenting with known or suspected heart failure should be approached in a systematic head-to-toe manner and is summarized in **Table 1**.

General

First, the patient should be assessed for general appearance; does the patient seem stable or unstable? Vital signs should be completed as with any encounter, specifically blood pressure, heart rate, respiratory rate, and oxygen saturation. Tachycardia may be indicative of heart failure, especially if decompensated, as it is a mechanism for the heart to compensate for both reduced stroke volume and cardiac output.[12] Hypotension during hospitalization for acute heart failure has been associated with poor short-term outcomes.[13]

Neck

Examination of the neck should be performed to evaluate the JVP (see "Special Maneuvers" below). Testing for hepatojugular reflux is another maneuver that can be performed and is indicative of ventricular dysfunction when present (see "Special Maneuvers" below).

Pulmonary

The pulmonary examination is a vital component in the assessment of heart failure as it can provide information on both the patient's respiratory and volume status. The examiner should auscultate the lungs for crackles, which may indicate the presence

Table 1 Summary of the physical examination assessment for heart failure	
System	**Examination**
General	Appearance Vitals
Neck	Jugular venous pressure Assessment for hepatojugular reflux (or abdominojugular test)
Pulmonary	Auscultation for: Crackles Diminished breath sounds Wheezing
Cardiac	Palpation for PMI Auscultation for cardiac murmurs and/or S3
Abdomen	Assessment for hepatomegaly and ascites
Extremities	Evaluate for edema, pulses, and coolness of extremities

of pulmonary edema as well as for diminished breath sounds which may indicate the presence of pleural effusion(s). Wheezing from heart failure may be heard during either inspiration or expiration. The term "cardiac asthma" has been used to refer to wheezing and coughing associated with heart failure and is thought to be secondary to pulmonary edema and pulmonary vascular congestion.[6,12,14]

Cardiac

Examination of the precordium includes the observation of the chest wall and palpation of the point of maximal impulse (PMI). The PMI is typically palpated at the 5th intercostal space in the mid-clavicular line, but is shifted laterally in dilated cardiomyopathy.[15] As the pads of the fingers are more sensitive than the fingertips, it is generally recommended that the finger pads be used when palpating the PMI. (See Video 1 for a demonstration on locating and assessing the cardiac PMI.)

During cardiac auscultation, attention should be paid to any cardiac murmurs, which can indicate valvular pathology as the potential etiology of heart failure as well as, vice versa, the functional result of dilatation of the heart from various cardiomyopathies. An "extra" heart sound (S3 or S4) can provide additional information. An S3 heart sound may be heard in patients with ventricular dysfunction and elevated left-sided ventricular filling pressures.[16] The S3 heart sound is very specific but has low sensitivity in systolic heart failure[12] (**Table 2**). Of note, an S3 heart sound is less frequently heard in patients prescribed beta-blocker medications.[15,17] An S4 heart sound may be heard in patients with heart failure and left ventricular hypertrophy.[12]

Abdomen

The abdominal examination includes the assessment of liver size, as hepatomegaly may occur due to congestion in the hepatic veins from right-sided heart failure.[12] If the patient reports increased abdominal girth or if bulging flanks are noted on examination, the examiner should consider performing maneuvers to assess for the presence of ascites due to right heart failure. These maneuvers include palpating for a

Table 2
Sensitivity, specificity, and likelihood ratios for physical examination findings in detecting left ventricular dysfunction - HFrEF

Finding	Sensitivity (%)	Specificity (%)	Likelihood Ratio Finding Present	Finding Absent
Abnormal Valsalva Response[30]	69–88	90–91	7.6	0.3
Crackles[25]	29	77	1.3	0.9
Elevated JVP[25]	24	99	27.0	0.8
Positive HJR[25]	33	94	6.0	0.7
S3 gallop[30]	11–51	85–98	3.4	0.7
S4 gallop[30]	31–67	55–68	Not significant	Not significant
Displaced Cardiac Apex[25]	66	95	16.0	0.4
Murmur of Mitral Regurgitation[30]	25	89	Not significant	Not significant
Hepatomegaly[30]	3	97	Not significant	Not significant
Dependent Edema[30]	20	86	1.4	0.9

*modified from Steve McGee's Evidence-Based Physical Diagnosis[30] and AAFP Diagnosis of Heart Failure in Adults[25].

fluid wave, percussion for flank dullness, and for shifting dullness. Though ascites is not commonly caused by heart failure (approximately 5% of cases),[18] it can occur due to liver congestion with resulting portal hypertension.[19]

Extremities

The extremities should be examined for pitting edema, which is a common sign of heart failure and fluid overload (as opposed to nonpitting edema which is often due to lymphedema). Pitting edema is an indicator of increased extracellular volume, but may also be found in other conditions aside from heart failure, such as renal and hepatic disease as well as chronic venous stasis and is therefore a helpful but nonspecific physical finding in heart failure. Diminished peripheral pulses and cool extremities are both signs of decreased circulation and may indicate severe decompensated heart failure and cardiogenic shock.

Special Maneuvers

If congestive heart failure is suspected based on the patient history and the above described general physical examination, the following maneuvers may be performed to further guide diagnosis and/or treatment. These maneuvers are also summarized in **Table 3**.

Jugular Venous Pressure

JVP is an approximation of right atrial pressure[20] and an indirect measurement of central venous pressure which can be estimated on physical examination by the inspection of the internal jugular vein in the neck. A normal JVP is 6 to 8 cm H2O above the right atrium.[21] Elevated JVP ($\geq$10 cm H2O) is the most useful finding for assessing ventricular filling pressures.[22,23] When present, it is indicative of volume overload and may guide further medical management, such as the adjustment of the dose and frequency of diuretic medications.

Measurement of JVP is performed with the examiner standing to the patient's right and assessing the right internal jugular venous pulse. The JVP will have a biphasic waveform in which a double pulsation is seen for each cardiac cycle, as opposed to the carotid artery which has a single pulsation per cardiac cycle. If there is difficulty visualizing the internal jugular waveform, assessment of the external jugular vein may also be used as an estimate of JVP.[6] However, the internal jugular is generally preferable as it is in direct connection with the superior vena cava and the right atrium. The examination may also be performed on the patient's left neck if the right is difficult to visualize (due to jugular vein thrombosis or the presence of a central venous catheter); however, the right internal jugular is preferred given its more direct line to the superior vena cava and thus the right atrium.[21]

When measuring JVP, the patient should be reclined at approximately 45° of elevation in the hospital bed or on the clinic room examination table with the neck slightly extended, head turned away from the examiner and chin tilted slightly upward. Using tangential lighting with a penlight or other bright light source pointed across the neck from anterior to posterior in direction, the examiner should visualize the double waveform pulsation of the JVP that reflects the pressure changes of the right atrium. Another useful method is to shine the light tangentially across the skin from anterior to posterior in a room with dim lighting to cast a shadow on the bedsheet; this may facilitate the visualization of vein motion.[24] The head of bed should be lowered until the top of the waveform of the internal jugular pulsation ("venous meniscus") is seen about halfway up the neck (this should be with the head of bed between a 0° and

Table 3
Summary of special physical examination maneuvers for heart failure

	Normal Result	Positive Finding
Jugular Venous Pressure (JVP)	6–8 cm H2O above the right atrium	≥ 10 cm H2O above the right atrium
Hepatojugular Reflux (HJR)	JVP elevation of 1–3 cm	Sustained (>10–15 s) increase of JVP > 4 cm
Valsalva Maneuver	Korotkoff sounds in phases I & IV	Korotkoff sounds in phase I ± phase II

90° angle from the horizontal axis). The venous meniscus is used to measure and calculate the JVP.

To measure the JVP, the top of the waveform of the internal jugular venous pulsation is used. A horizontal line (parallel to the floor) is then envisioned from this point and also a separate horizontal line is envisioned from the level of the sternal angle. The vertical distance between these 2 points is then measured in centimeters and added to the distance between the sternal angle and right atrium (which is estimated to be 5 cm) to determine the JVP (**Fig. 1**).

Elevated JVP has a high specificity (90%) but low sensitivity (30%) in determining elevated left ventricular filling.[12] Though locating and estimating the JVP is one of the most challenging aspects of the entire physical examination, if it is elevated, it has a high positive likelihood ratio (LR) of 27 in the detection of left ventricular dysfunction and thus is a very useful finding for diagnosing heart failure.[25]

A common pitfall in evaluating the JVP is to mistake the carotid artery for the internal jugular vein. While the carotid upstroke only has a single pulsation as compared with 2 for the JVP, another method to differentiate them is to apply pressure 1 to 2 inches below the impulse. If the pulsation remains visible then it is the carotid artery, but if it disappears with pressure below the impulse then it is the jugular vein. Another technique is to apply pressure to the right upper quadrant of the abdomen. In most patients, the JVP will rise initially with this increased abdominal pressure, while the carotid pulsation will remain the same without changing in location.[6] (See Video 2 for a demonstration of locating the internal jugular vein.)

If heart failure is present, the examination for JVP may need to take place with the patient in the fully upright position as the JVP may be so elevated that it is not visible at 45° elevation. Similarly, if heart failure is not present or if the patient's heart failure is well controlled, the head of the bed may need to be lowered below 45° to visualize the JVP. A common mistake for the novice examiner to make is to fail to adjust the examination table or bed control elevation to best accentuate the JVP.

Hepatojugular Reflux and Abdominojugular Test

Checking for hepatojugular reflux is another adjunctive physical examination maneuver in assessing the JVP for physical examination evidence of congestive heart failure.[26] This test is done with the patient in the supine position with the head of bed raised to a 30° to 45° angle. After visualizing the JVP, mild to moderate pressure (20–35 mm Hg) is applied to the right upper quadrant or the middle of the abdomen for 30 to 60 seconds,[12,27] which increases venous return to the heart. In the presence of heart failure, the right ventricle is unable to adjust to the increased blood volume, which is reflected in an increase in JVP.[26]

A positive HJR is considered to be an increase in the JVP 4 cm or greater and sustained for at least 10 to 15 seconds when abdominal pressure is applied and a subsequent decrease in JVP after pressure is released.[6,26,28] HJR is indicative of ventricular dysfunction, which may be right, left or both ventricles in origin. In the absence of right ventricular or mitral valve pathology, a positive HJR is suggestive of elevated left ventricular pressure and predicts a PCWP of greater than 15 mm Hg.[26]

The abdominojugular test involves exerting pressure in the epigastrium with the same intensity and length of time and is believed to cause similar pathophysiologic changes in the patient with heart failure (see Video 3 for demonstration). Either HJR or the abdominojugular test can be performed but it is not necessary to use both techniques.

Valsalva Maneuver

The Valsalva maneuver is useful for assessing for elevated left-sided filling pressures and is a predictor of elevated PCWP.[6] Though it is rarely used in clinical practice (likely due to a lack of physician familiarity with the technique), it has reasonable specificity of 91% and sensitivity of 69% for the presence of heart failure.[12]

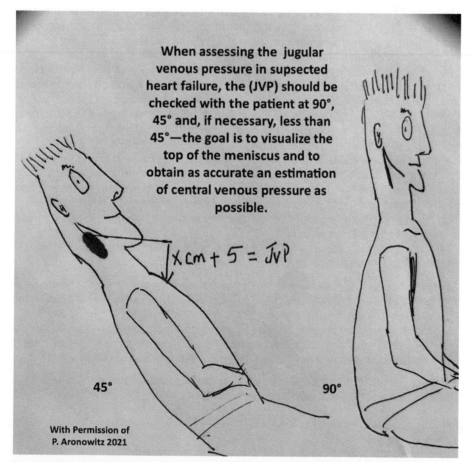

Fig. 1. When assessing the jugular venous pressure in suspected heart failure, the (JVP) should be checked with the patient at 90, 45° and, if necessary, less than 45°

Table 4
Phases of the Valsalva maneuver

	Korotkoff Sounds	
Phase	**Normal**	**Congestive Heart Failure**
I (Onset of strain)	Present	Present
II (Maintenance of strain)	Absent	Present OR Absent
III (Release of strain)	Absent	Absent
IV (After release of strain)	Present	Absent

To perform the Valsalva maneuver in assessing for the presence of heart failure the patient's baseline blood pressure is first measured. Next, the blood pressure cuff is inflated to 15 mm Hg above the systolic blood pressure. While auscultating over the brachial artery, the patient is asked to bear down (forced expiration against a closed glottis).[29]

There are 4 phases with the Valsalva maneuver which correspond to the following findings in **Table 4**.

In *phase I*, the onset of strain, there is a transient increase in systolic blood pressure due to the emptying of blood from the pulmonary veins and Korotkoff sounds are heard in both the healthy patient and patient with heart failure.[12]

In *phase II*, the maintenance of strain, an increase in intrathoracic pressure leads to a decrease in venous return and cardiac preload. In the healthy patient, the blood pressure decreases during this phase back to baseline and Korotkoff sounds are no longer heard.[12] However, in patients with heart failure, there may not be a decrease in blood pressure during this phase because the left ventricle remains filled due to elevated left ventricular pressures before straining.[6] Therefore, Korotkoff sounds may be present or absent in phase II for patients with heart failure.

In *phase III*, the release of strain, healthy individuals respond with an overshoot of blood pressure above baseline (*phase IV*) due to the return of normal venous blood flow to the heart and Korotkoff sounds are heard again.[12,29] In the healthy patient, Korotkoff sounds are heard in both phase I and IV.[30] In the patient with heart failure, Korotkoff sounds are not heard in phase IV due to the inability of the heart to respond with an increase in the cardiac output.

To summarize, in patients with congestive heart failure, there are 2 potentially abnormal Valsalva responses[30]:

1. *Korotkoff sounds are only present in phase I.* Korotkoff sounds do not reappear in phase IV because the heart is unable to increase cardiac output to respond to the blood pressure decrease in phase II.[30]
2. *Korotkoff sounds are present in phases I and II.* Korotkoff sounds remain in phase II but are not present in phases III and IV. This is hypothesized to occur due to increased volume maintaining blood supply to the right and left heart.[30]

It is important to note that the use of beta-blocking medications may result in a false-positive result by preventing the phase IV overshoot of blood pressure.[30]

DISCUSSION

As previously mentioned, the physical examination is helpful to the examiner in determining the diagnosis of heart failure and for subsequently monitoring treatment effects.

To maximize the utility of the physical examination, it is important to recognize the relevance of each clinical finding when considering the diagnosis of heart failure. **Table 2** provides information on the sensitivity, specificity, and LR of the physical examination findings discussed in this article. Having knowledge of these values allows for a better understanding of the posttest probability of heart failure as a diagnosis based on a combination of known prevalence of heart failure in the population being assessed, examination findings and their positive and negative LR and the pretest probability of heart failure based on the clinical history obtained.

As noted in **Table 2**, of the numerous examination findings that may be present in heart failure, the Valsalva maneuver has one of the better combinations of sensitivity, specificity, and positive and negative LR, but is rarely checked.[12] Given these values, it may be judicious to use this examination maneuver when there is the question of the diagnosis of heart failure. A displaced cardiac apex on examination is also useful in the diagnosis of congestive heart failure with a high positive LR when the finding is present and is the most accurate predictor of reduced EF.[31]

In addition to guiding diagnosis and treatment, the physical examination can also provide important prognostic information. For example, an elevated JVP has been found to be associated with an increased risk of hospitalization for heart failure, progression of heart failure, and death from all causes.[17] A study examining over 2000 patients admitted for acute heart failure found an association between elevated JVP and an increase in short- and long-term mortality.[23] Similarly, the presence of a third heart sound (S3 gallop) with or without an elevated jugular venous pressure has been found to be associated with progression of heart failure as well as an increased risk of death from all causes.[17] The presence of HJR is also clinically significant in hospitalized patients as it is an important prognostic indicator for postdischarge outcomes. Patients with persistent HJR on discharge were noted to have a higher 6-month mortality based on the data from the ESCAPE trial.[26]

Understanding the prognostic implications of the physical examination findings found in patients with heart failure can identify patients who may need more cautious and frequent follow-up after hospital discharge.

CLINICS CARE POINTS

- Bendopnea is a symptom recently described in heart failure in which patients have shortness of breath while bending forward.[11]

- To assess for jugular venous pressure in heart failure, the clinician should examine the patient in the upright position to exclude a markedly elevated JVP which may be missed if the patient is not adequately elevated.

- When examining JVP, a common pitfall is to mistake the carotid artery for the internal jugular vein. There are several methods to distinguish between the 2[6]. The carotid pulsation has a single pulsation, does not disappear with proximal compression, and does not increase in height when checking for the presence of hepatojugular reflux.

- Elevated JVP has been found to be associated with increased short- and long-term mortality in patients hospitalized for acute heart failure.[23]

- The Valsalva maneuver has one of the best combinations of sensitivity, specificity, and LR for diagnosing heart failure but is an underused examination maneuver.

- Recent eye surgery and acute coronary ischemia are contraindications to the Valsalva maneuver as it increases intraocular pressure and there have also been reported arrhythmias with the maneuver.[27,30]

- When the Valsalva maneuver is performed on a healthy patient, Korotkoff sounds are heard in phase I (onset of strain) and phase IV (after the release of strain).
- When the Valsalva maneuver is performed on a patient with congestive heart failure, there are 2 potential abnormal responses[30]:
  1. Korotkoff sounds in phase I only (onset of strain)
  2. Korotkoff sounds in phase I (onset of strain) and II (maintenance of strain) only
- Use of a beta-blocker may result in a false-positive result with the Valsalva maneuver by preventing the phase IV overshoot of blood pressure.[30] Use of beta-blockers may also result in a false negative S3 heart sound.
- The presence of hepatojugular reflux on discharge in patients hospitalized for heart failure is associated with an increase in 6-month mortality[26]

SUMMARY

The clinical examination continues to be very important in the assessment and management of congestive heart failure and provides useful and cost-effective information which can then be used to guide more extensive as well as expensive diagnostic imaging and laboratory testing. Patients with heart failure may present with a variety of symptoms. Classic symptoms include dyspnea, PND, orthopnea, edema, and weight gain, but symptoms may also be nonspecific such as fatigue and anorexia. The physical examination can help guide the need for further workup, particularly when there is a general understanding of the positive and negative likelihood ratios for various physical findings and examination maneuvers.

It is recommended that the initial examination in the patient with shortness of breath be approached in a head-to-toe manner and special maneuvers such as the measurement of the JVP, Valsalva maneuver, and hepatojugular reflux done as needed when there is suspicion for heart failure. These physical examination findings not only assist with diagnosis and treatment but also have prognostic implications for hospitalized patients.

Despite physician inclination to frequently jump directly to costly diagnostic testing for the diagnosis and evaluation of heart failure, this article has demonstrated the continued utility of a disease-based physical examination for heart failure.

Supplementary data to this article can be found online at https://doi.org/10.1016/j.mcna.2021.12.002.

DISCLOSURE

The authors have nothing to disclose.

SUPPLEMENTARY DATA

Supplementary data related to this article can be found online at https://doi.org/10.1016/j.mcna.2021.12.002.

REFERENCES

1. Ambrosy AP, Fonarow GC, Butler J, et al. The global health and economic burden of hospitalizations for heart failure: lessons learned from hospitalized heart failure registries. J Am Coll Cardiol 2014;63(12):1123–33.
2. Virani SS, Alonso A, Aparicio HJ, et al. Heart Disease and Stroke Statistics-2021 Update: A Report From the American Heart Association. Circulation 2021;143(8):e254–743.

3. McCullough PA, Philbin EF, Spertus JA, et al. Confirmation of a heart failure epidemic: findings from the Resource Utilization Among Congestive Heart Failure (REACH) study. J Am Coll Cardiol 2002;39(1):60–9.

4. Caldentey G, Khairy P, Roy D, et al. Prognostic value of the physical examination in patients with heart failure and atrial fibrillation. JACC: Heart Fail 2014;2(1): 15–23.

5. Leier CV, Chatterjee K. The physical examination in heart failure–Part I. Congest Heart Fail 2007;13(1):41–7.

6. Thibodeau JT, Drazner MH. The role of the clinical examination in patients with heart failure. JACC: Heart Fail 2018;6(7):543–51.

7. Leier CV, Chatterjee K. The physical examination in Heart Failure?Part II. Congest Heart Fail 2007;13(2):99–0103.

8. Felker GM, Anstrom KJ, Adams KF, et al. Effect of Natriuretic Peptide-Guided Therapy on Hospitalization or Cardiovascular Mortality in High-Risk Patients With Heart Failure and Reduced Ejection Fraction: A Randomized Clinical Trial. JAMA 2017;318(8):713–20.

9. Ponikowski P, Voors AA, Anker SD, et al. 2016 ESC Guidelines for the diagnosis and treatment of acute and chronic heart failure: The Task Force for the diagnosis and treatment of acute and chronic heart failure of the European Society of Cardiology (ESC)Developed with the special contribution of the Heart Failure Association (HFA) of the ESC [published correction appears in Eur Heart J. 2016 Dec 30. Eur Heart J 2016;37(27):2129–200.

10. Mukerji V. Dyspnea, Orthopnea, and Paroxysmal Nocturnal Dyspnea. In: Walker HK, Hall WD, Hurst JW, editors. Clinical methods: the history, physical, and laboratory examinations. 3rd edition. Boston: Butterworths; 1990. p. 78–80. Available at: https://www.ncbi.nlm.nih.gov/books/NBK213/.

11. Thibodeau JT, Turer AT, Gualano SK, et al. Characterization of a novel symptom of advanced heart failure: bendopnea. JACC Heart Fail 2014;2(1):24–31.

12. Shamsham F, Mitchell J. Essentials of the diagnosis of heart failure. Am Fam Physician 2000;61(5):1319–28.

13. Patel PA, Heizer G, O'Connor CM, et al. Hypotension during hospitalization for acute heart failure is independently associated with 30-day mortality: findings from ASCEND-HF. Circ Heart Fail 2014;7(6):918–25.

14. Tanabe T, Rozycki HJ, Kanoh S, et al. Cardiac asthma: new insights into an old disease. Expert Rev Respir Med 2012;6(6):705–14.

15. Damy T, Kallvikbacka-Bennett A, Zhang J, et al. Does the physical examination still have a role in patients with suspected heart failure? Eur J Heart Fail 2011; 13(12):1340–8.

16. Collins SP, Peacock WF, Lindsell CJ, et al. S3 detection as a diagnostic and prognostic aid in emergency department patients with acute dyspnea. Ann Emerg Med 2009;53(6):748–57.

17. Drazner MH, Rame JE, Stevenson LW, et al. Prognostic importance of elevated jugular venous pressure and a third heart sound in patients with heart failure. N Engl J Med 2001;345(8):574–81.

18. Aisenberg GM. Peritoneal catheter for massive cardiac ascites. BMJ Case Rep 2013;2013. bcr2013008992.

19. Christou L, Economou M, Economou G, et al. Characteristics of ascitic fluid in cardiac ascites. Scand J Gastroenterol 2007;42(9):1102–5.

20. Drazner MH, Hellkamp AS, Leier CV, et al. Value of clinician assessment of hemodynamics in advanced heart failure: the ESCAPE trial. Circ Heart Fail 2008;1(3): 170–7.

21. Applefeld MM. The Jugular Venous Pressure and Pulse Contour. In: Walker HK, Hall WD, Hurst JW, editors. Clinical methods: the history, physical, and laboratory examinations. 3rd edition. Boston: Butterworths; 1990. Chapter 19. Available at: https://www.ncbi.nlm.nih.gov/books/NBK300/. Accessed July 23, 2021.

22. Cohn JN. Jugular venous pressure monitoring: A lost art? J Card Fail 1997; 3(2):71–3.

23. Chernomordik F, Berkovitch A, Schwammenthal E, et al. Short- and Long-Term Prognostic Implications of Jugular Venous Distension in Patients Hospitalized With Acute Heart Failure. Am J Cardiol 2016;118(2):226–31.

24. Chua Chiaco JM, Parikh NI, Fergusson DJ. The jugular venous pressure revisited. Cleve Clin J Med 2013;80(10):638–44.

25. Dosh SA. Diagnosis of heart failure in adults. Am Fam Physician 2004;70(11): 2145–52.

26. Omar HR, Guglin M. Clinical and Prognostic Significance of Positive Hepatojugular Reflux on Discharge in Acute Heart Failure: Insights from the ESCAPE Trial. Biomed Res Int 2017;2017:5734749.

27. Vaidya Y, Bhatti H, Dhamoon AS. Hepatojugular Reflux. In: StatPearls. Treasure Island (FL): StatPearls Publishing; 2021. Available at: https://www.ncbi.nlm.nih.gov/books/NBK526097/. Accessed July 21, 2021.

28. McGee Steven. Inspection of the Neck Veins. In: Evidence-based physical diagnosis. 3rd edition. Philadelphia, (PA): Elsevier – Health Science; 2012. p. 293–306.

29. Srivastav S, Jamil RT, Zeltser R. Valsalva Maneuver. In: StatPearls. Treasure Island (FL): StatPearls Publishing; 2021. Available at: https://www.ncbi.nlm.nih.gov/books/NBK537248/. Accessed July 21, 2021.

30. McGee Steven. Congestive Heart Failure. In: Evidence-based physical diagnosis. 3rd edition. Philadelphia, (PA): Elsevier – Health Science; 2012. p. 405–12.

31. Davie AP, Francis CM, Caruana L, et al. Assessing diagnosis in heart failure: which features are any use? QJM 1997;90(5):335–9.

Delirium

Craig R. Keenan, MD[a],*, Sharad Jain, MD[b]

KEYWORDS

- Delirium • Confusion • Assessment • Examination • Attention • CAM • Cognition

KEY POINTS

- Delirium is a common neuropsychiatric disorder that can be a harbinger of serious underlying conditions, yet it is often underrecognized.
- There are validated tools using the clinician's history and physical examination that have high sensitivity and specificity that should be used to diagnose delirium.
- Diagnosing the underlying cause of delirium is also a critical step in the patient's care. Physical examination as a tool to find these underlying causes is not well studied, but still can provide important clues to the clinician.

INTRODUCTION/DEFINITIONS/BACKGROUND

Delirium is a very common neuropsychiatric condition affecting medical patients. The most commonly used definition of delirium is outlined in the *Diagnostic and Statistical Manual of Mental Disorders, Fifth Edition* (DSM-V), and has the following criteria[1]:

- Disturbance in attention (ie, reduced ability to direct, focus, sustain, and shift attention) and awareness.
- Change in cognition (eg, memory deficit, disorientation, language disturbance, perceptual disturbance) that is not explained by a preexisting, established, or evolving dementia.
- The disturbance develops over a short period (usually hours to days) and tends to fluctuate during the course of the day.
- There is evidence from the history, physical examination, or laboratory findings *that the disturbance is caused by a direct physiologic consequence of a general medical condition, an intoxicating substance, medication use, or more than one cause.*

The estimated prevalence of delirium is 23% of hospitalized adults, 4% to 38% of patients in the nursing home, 35% of patients in palliative care settings, and 8% to

[a] University of California, Davis School of Medicine, 4150 V Street, Suite 1100, Sacramento, California 95817, USA; [b] University of California, Davis School of Medicine, 4610 X Street, Suite 4202, Sacramento, California 95817, USA
* Corresponding author.
E-mail address: crkeenan@ucdavis.edu

Med Clin N Am 106 (2022) 459–469
https://doi.org/10.1016/j.mcna.2021.12.003
0025-7125/22/© 2022 Elsevier Inc. All rights reserved.

17% of patients in emergency department settings. The prevalence is particularly high in patients in the intensive care unit (ICU) at 32%, with a 50% to 70% prevalence in mechanically ventilated patients. Last, delirium is a common complication of surgery in older adults with an incidence of 15% to 25% after major elective surgery and up to 50% after higher risk surgeries.[2–4]

Despite these high prevalence rates, delirium often goes unrecognized by clinicians, with up to 65% to 88% of cases not identified by clinicians when compared with formal assessments.[3] One reason for this observation is that only 25% of delirium is the so-called hyperactive delirium, which is characterized by agitation and is more easily identified. Up to 75% of cases in older adults are the more quiet, hypoactive delirium, which often goes unrecognized.[4]

Often delirium is a signal of underlying potentially dangerous and treatable conditions, so it is critical to recognize and address it. The presence of delirium in patients portends a worse prognosis, with increased mortality, impaired physical functioning, incident dementia, and institutionalization; it also is a risk factor for medical complications, increased length of hospital stay, and discharge to post–acute care nursing facilities.[4] Last, delirium can have a highly variable course, lasting a few days in some patients but causing identifiable cognitive dysfunction for many months after the initial diagnosis.

Using the DSM-V definition of delirium, one can outline 2 steps that must be undertaken by the clinician to make a complete diagnosis of delirium. The first step is to identify both the characteristic disturbance in attention and change in cognition. Although the history is very important, there are mental status examinations that can help to identify the cognitive and attention deficits. The second step is to identify the underlying medical cause of the disturbance, whether a medical condition or a reaction to a medication or substance. Here, again, the history is paramount, but the physical examination can provide many clues to underlying conditions at the root of a delirious state.

DISCUSSION
Diagnosis of Delirium

Our literature review did not find any studies that specifically evaluated the physical examination or specific physical examination maneuvers in the diagnosis of delirium. There are, however, many studies of diagnostic and severity assessment tools for delirium that incorporate both the history and mental status examination—the mental status examination being an essential part of the physical examination in all physical examination texts. These tools are a crucial first step in diagnosing delirium. A 2010 systematic review of these diagnostic instruments found that, for hospitalized, non-ICU patients, the Confusion Assessment Method (CAM) yielded the best test characteristics.[5] The CAM was first published in 1990 and has been validated in many different settings (**Box 1**).[6] The CAM instrument prompts the assessing clinician to answer 9 questions to assess mental status, takes about 5 minutes to complete, and uses history from the patient, care team, and family together with the clinician's assessments on mental status examination to identify the attention and cognitive deficits. In the original CAM study, the geriatricians used the Mini Mental Status Examination to assess cognition, but other tools such as the MiniCog or the Montreal Cognitive Assessment can be used. These tests are then used to complete the CAM diagnostic algorithm that assesses 4 features for diagnosis. **Box 1** outlines the CAM diagnostic algorithm. To diagnose delirium, the patient must have (1) acute change or a fluctuating course (Feature 1) *and* inattention (Feature 2) *plus one of either* disorganized thinking (Feature 3) or altered level of consciousness (Feature 4).

> **Box 1**
> **The confusion assessment method diagnostic tool[6]**
>
> Feature 1: Acute onset and fluctuating course
>
> Feature 2: Inattention
>
> Feature 3: Disorganized thinking
>
> Feature 4: Altered level of consciousness
>
> The diagnosis of delirium requires the presence of both 1 and 2, and either 3 or 4.
>
> Inouye SK, van Dyck CH, Alessi CA, et al. Clarifying confusion: the confusion assessment method. Ann Intern Med 1990;113:941.

Real world use of the CAM instrument often uses assessments during routine care by physicians and nurses, as opposed to formal interviews and cognitive assessments by geriatricians or researchers. This use of more routine care assessment reduces the CAM's sensitivity to as low as 19% in one study of nurse assessments compared with those made by formal researchers.[7] The amount of time required to administer the CAM also limits its clinical use by busy clinicians. Over the years, other CAM-based instruments that are shorter have been developed and studied that incorporate brief but standardized mental status testing for clinicians, which increases the sensitivity. The test characteristics for each of these instruments are outlined in **Table 1**.

The 3-Minute Diagnostic Interview for Delirium Using the Confusion Assessment Method (3D-CAM) is designed for use with general medical patients. The 3D-CAM consists of 20 items in total, 10 of which are administered directly to patients, including 7 items assessing orientation and attention and 3 items assessing patient symptoms. The other 10 items are observations to assess the 4 CAM diagnostic features and are completed by the assessor at the conclusion of the interview. With training, the 3D-CAM can be completed in 3 minutes or less. A "skip" pattern method of delivering the 3D-CAM allows the clinician to skip some of the 20 items once there is a "positive" answer in each CAM feature. This approach can further reduce the 3D-CAM assessment time. The 3D-CAM has excellent testing characteristics, with a high sensitivity and specificity, making it a useful clinical diagnostic tool.

Table 1
Characteristics of diagnostic tools for delirium

Tool	Sensitivity (%)	Specificity (%)	Likelihood Ratio Positive	Likelihood Ratio Negative
CAM[5]	86	93	9.6	0.16
3D-CAM[8]	95	94	15.8	0.05
CAM-ICU[10]	85	95	15.5	0.16
bCAM[11]	84	96	19.9	0.17
4AT[13]	88	88	7.3	0.14
Ultrabrief 2-Item Screen (UB-2)[14]	93	64	2.6	0.11

Abbreviations: 3D-CAM, 3-Minute Diagnostic Interview for Delirium Using the Confusion Assessment Method; bCAM, Brief Confusion Assessment Method; CAM-ICU, Confusion Assessment Method for the Intensive Care Unit; UB-2, UltraBrief 2-Item Screen.
Data from Refs.[5,8,10,11,13,14]

The Confusion Assessment Method for the Intensive Care Unit (CAM-ICU) uses the commonly used Glasgow Coma Scale or Richmond Agitation Sedation Scale (RASS) to assess fluctuation in condition and altered level of consciousness. CAM-ICU also includes tests that can be done in nonverbal intubated patient, using either picture recognition or the Vigilance A Random Letter Test to assess attentiveness.[9] The CAM-ICU has been validated in multiple studies and has high sensitivity (85%) and specificity (95%).[10]

The Brief Confusion Assessment Method (bCAM) has been studied in patients in the emergency department; it uses the RASS for level of consciousness, asks the patient to recite months of the year backward to assess attention, and has the patient answer a series of simple questions and follow a simple motor commands to assess for disorganized thinking. bCAM also has excellent sensitivity and specificity when used in the emergency department.[11]

In addition, the non-CAM based 4AT test is also widely used and well studied.[12,13] This test scores patients on 4 items, is easy to administer, does not require training, and takes less than 2 minutes to complete. The assessor asks the patient to recite the months of the year backward to assess attention and asks the patient 4 questions (age, date of birth, current place, and year) to assess cognition. The clinician then assesses for alertness and any acute change and/or fluctuation in condition. A recent meta-analysis of multiple studies showed 88% sensitivity and specificity.[13]

All these newer instruments are quick to administer and have excellent test characteristics with both low negative likelihood ratio (LR) and high positive LR. These instruments are helpful in both diagnosing and ruling out delirium when used in the appropriate patients.

Even with these shorter instruments, busy clinicians are not always able to perform them in all patients in whom delirium may be occurring, leading to missed opportunities to diagnose this disorder. A reasonable approach is to focus the use of these instruments to confirm delirium in suspected cases (the patient reported to be mildly confused overnight or difficult to arouse in the morning), or to find cases in high-risk patients (the patient with underlying dementia, recent major surgery, or ICU admission). For busy clinicians, it would also be ideal to have a quick screening tool for delirium that could be used in nearly all patients. Fick and colleagues[14] assessed the individual items in the 3D-CAM to try to find 1- or 2-item screens to identify delirium quickly. The single-item screen "Recite the months of the year backward" had a sensitivity of 83% and specificity of 69%, with corresponding LR+ of 2.7 and LR− of 0.24. The 2-item combination that worked the best was (1) "Recite the months of the year backward" and (2) "What is the day of the week?" This combination of these 2 items had a sensitivity of 93% and specificity of 64%, with corresponding LR+ of 2.6 and LR− of 0.11; this is now called the UltraBrief 2-Item Screen (UB-2).[14] As a negative screen, this tool is very good to rule out delirium. However, the low LR+ requires that a positive screen be followed up by a more in-depth assessment to confirm the diagnosis of delirium.

The creators of the 3D-CAM and UB-2 have combined these results into a single, 1-page instrument called the UB-CAM (Fig. 1)[15]; it starts with the 2-item screen and, if either are positive, moves the clinician through the remaining portions of the 3D-CAM for more specificity. A study comparing different screening algorithms using these tools found that using the UB-CAM took only an average of 1 minute 14 seconds when the 2-item screen was positive and then followed up with a 3D-CAM using the "skip" method of questions.[16] The UB-CAM tool can easily be implemented in a busy clinical practice for general medical patients.

Ultra-Brief CAM [UB-CAM] UB-2/3D-CAM	
Instructions: Administer items in order specified. Direct questions of patients are *shown in italics*. • A positive sign for delirium is any incorrect, don't know, non-response, or non-sensical response. • CAM features 1-4 are indicated with F1, F2, F3, F4, respectively.	
Severe lethargy or severe altered level of consciousness	Check
1 **Severe lethargy or severe altered level of consciousness (no or minimal response to voice/touch).** If present, terminate assessment and ratings. **Patient is considered DELIRIOUS.** If not present, proceed to UB-2 Screener.	☐
UB-2 Screener	Check if sign positive
2 **Ask both questions**	
Please tell me the day of the week (F3)	☐
Please tell me months of the year backwards, say "December" as your first month (F2)	☐
Checkpoint: - If neither sign is positive/checked, STOP: patient is NOT DELIRIOUS - If at least one sign is positive/checked, proceed to next section (3) and follow as directed	
3D-CAM Algorithm: Part 1 - Patient Assessment	
3 **Assess Disorganized Thinking (Feature 3/F3). Stop, and go to Section 4, after the first positive sign (error) of Disorganized Thinking. Carry-forward errors from the UB2 Screener:**	Check if sign positive
Carry forward: Was the patient unable to correctly identify the day of the week? (F3, UB2)	☐
Please tell me the year we are in right now (F3)	☐
Please tell me what type of place is this [hospital, rehab, home, etc.] (F3)	☐
4 **Assess Attention (Feature 2/F2). Stop, and go to Section 5, after the first positive sign (error) of Inattention. Carry-forward errors from the UB2 Screener:**	Check if sign positive
Carry forward: Was the patient unable to correctly name the months of the year backwards (UB2)	☐
Please tell me the days of the week backwards, say "Saturday" as your first day(F2)	☐
Repeat these numbers in backwards order: "7-5-1" (F2)	☐
Repeat these numbers in backwards order: "8-2-4-3" (F2)	☐
5 **Assess Acute change or Fluctuation (Feature 1/F1). Stop, and go to Section 6, after the first positive sign of Acute Change is noted:**	Check if sign positive
Over the past day have you felt confused? (F1)	☐
Over the past day did you think that you were not really in the hospital [or location of interview]? (F1)	☐
Over the past day did you see things that were not really there? (F1)	☐
3D-CAM Algorithm: Part 2 - Interviewer Ratings	
6 **Ratings for Altered Level of Consciousness (Feature 4/F4). Stop, and go to Section 7, after first sign of Altered Level of Consciousness.**	Check if sign positive
Was the patient sleepy during the interview? (requires that they actually fall asleep) (F4)	☐
Did the patient show hypervigilance? (F4)	☐
7 **Ratings for Disorganized Thinking (Feature 3/F3). Only rate if all of the patient assessment items for Feature 3 above were responded to correctly. Stop, and go to Section 8, after the first sign of Disorganized Thinking is noted.**	Check if sign positive
Was the patient's flow of ideas unclear or illogical? (F3)	☐
Was the patient's conversation rambling, inappropriately verbose, or tangential? (F3)	☐
Was the patient's speech unusually limited or sparse? (F3)	☐
8 **Ratings for Attention (Feature 2/F2). Only rate if all of the patient assessment items for Feature 2 above were responded to correctly. Stop, and go to Section 9, after first sign of Inattention is noted.**	Check if sign positive
Does the patient have trouble keeping track of what was said or following directions? (F2)	☐
Does the patient seem inappropriately distracted by external stimuli? (F2)	☐
9 **Ratings for Acute Change or Fluctuation (Feature 1/F1). Only rate if all patient assessment items for Feature 1 above were negative. Stop, and go to CAM Rating Summary, after 1st positive sign of Acute Change or Fluctuation is noted.**	Check if sign positive
Did the patient's level of consciousness, level of attention or speech/thinking fluctuate during the interview? (F1)	☐
If no prior assessments, is there evidence an acute change in memory or thinking according to records, or informant? (F1)	☐
If prior assessments, are there any new signs of delirium based on above questions (new errors, positive ratings)? (F1)	☐
Checkpoint: CAM Delirium feature assessment and rating summary	Check
- At least one sign of Acute Change and/or Fluctuation was noted (Feature 1)	☐
- At least one sign of Inattention was noted (Feature 2)	☐
- At least one sign of Disorganized Thinking was noted (Feature 3)	☐
- At least one sign of Altered Level of Consciousness was noted (Feature 4)	☐
CAM Criteria for Delirium: (Feature 1 AND Feature 2) AND (Feature 3 OR Feature 4) Is delirium present? Yes ☐ No ☐	

Fig. 1. Ultrabrief Confusion Assessment Method (UB-CAM).[15]

All these diagnostic tools are readily accessible by an Internet search. Several are also available on clinical decision tool applications for smartphones or as individual smartphone applications that can be downloaded.

Diagnosis of Underlying Causes of Delirium

Once the diagnosis of delirium is made, the second step is to determine the underlying cause. Although sometimes a single factor causes delirium, more often it has a multifactorial cause, especially in older patients. It is important to consider a broad differential diagnosis to determine underlying causes, especially those that can be addressed and potentially reversed.This will include a thorough history, which often requires collaboration with family members and nursing or other clinical staff to get a more complete history due to patient confusion. It is also critical to review the patient's medications, especially drugs that were recently started as well as any potential drug interactions. Sedative-hypnotic, analgesic, and anticholinergic medications are especially common culprits in causing delirium and should be discontinued or substituted whenever possible. Similarly, it is important to assess for substance use, as withdrawal and intoxication syndromes can contribute to delirium. The clinician should assess for any pain or discomfort that may result in delirium; common causes include thirst, urinary retention, and constipation. A thorough physical examination can also provide clues as to the cause, and is discussed further in the article. Last, patients will usually get targeted laboratory and other studies, based on the history and physical examination; this often includes assessing renal and liver function, electrolytes, complete blood cell count, thyroid studies, urinalysis, electrocardiogram, and targeted radiographic imaging, whether chest radiograph or computed tomography.

Table 2 lists the common causes for delirium and the possible physical examination findings associated with them. Although many of these causes require laboratory studies to confirm, the clinician can obtain significant information from the physical examination.

In performing the physical examination, the clinician should start by reviewing the patient's vital signs. An abnormal temperature (high or low) might suggest an infection, low blood pressure may indicate volume depletion or shock, high blood pressure could indicate hypertensive encephalopathy, and tachypnea might suggest metabolic acidosis, pneumonia, or pulmonary embolus. The remaining examination should look for clues to the precipitants of delirium. The head examination should look for evidence of trauma, which could be a clue to an underlying subdural hematoma. Examining for ophthalmoplegia could uncover a stroke, tumor, or Wernicke encephalopathy. The neck examination may reveal thyromegaly, which could be a clue for thyroid disease. Chest examination will look for evidence of consolidation (bronchial breath sounds, egophony, dullness to percussion) or reactive airways disease (wheezing, prolonged expiratory phase, accessory muscle use), whereas the cardiovascular examination will assess for signs of heart failure. Abdominal examination may give clues to an intra-abdominal infection such as appendicitis, diverticulitis, or cholecystitis. Careful observation and palpation of the abdomen can sometimes reveal abdominal distension or palpable stool burden revealing evidence of fecal impaction, which can also contribute to delirium in the elderly. Suprapubic palpation may reveal tenderness with a urinary tract infection or urinary retention. Percussion for bladder enlargement may also reveal bladder distension and urinary retention, which is a common contributor to delirium in the elderly (sometimes referred to as the "cystocerebral syndrome"). Careful evaluation of the skin in search of skin and soft tissue infections such as erysipelas, cellulitis, and infected pressure ulcers should be performed, especially on the feet, hip, and sacral and buttock regions. In addition to the mental status examination, a complete neurologic examination is warranted. Focal neurologic findings of an acute stroke or those suggestive of meningitis may be discovered, but there may also be clues to other diagnoses such as vitamin B_{12} deficiency (hyperreflexia due to myelopathy or sensory loss due to peripheral neuropathy).

Looking for signs of advanced chronic liver disease, such as decreased body hair, prominent abdominal wall veins, gynecomastia, spider angiomas, palmar erythema,

Table 2
Common causes of delirium

Causes	Physical Examination Findings
Metabolic abnormalities	
Hyponatremia/hypernatremia	
Hypercalcemia	
Hypoglycemia/hyperglycemia	
Hypercarbia	Asterixis
Hypoxemia	
Hypothyroidism	Delayed relaxation of ankle reflexes, pretibial edema, bradycardia, hypertension, dry skin, coarse voice
Hyperthyroidism	Fine tremor, proptosis, pretibial edema, eyelid lag, eyelid retraction, goiter, tachycardia
Vitamin B_{12} deficiency	Hyperreflexia, reduced sensation
Vitamin B_1 deficiency (Wernicke encephalopathy)	Ophthalmoplegia, confabulation
Adrenal insufficiency	Hyperpigmentation
Neurologic disorders	
Seizures	Tongue trauma
Subdural hematoma/head injury	Contusions, abrasions to scalp
Stroke	Focal neurologic findings
Hypertensive encephalopathy	
Systemic diseases	
Hepatic encephalopathy	Asterixis, ascites, spider angiomata, palmar erythema
Uremic encephalopathy	Asterixis, uremic frost
Acute pulmonary embolism	Tachycardia, parasternal heave, unilateral leg swelling
Acute myocardial ischemia	
Heart failure	Cardiomegaly, S3, S4, peripheral edema, elevated neck veins
Chronic obstructive pulmonary disease exacerbation	Wheezing, prolonged expiration, accessory muscle use, asterixis
Urinary retention	Enlarged bladder to palpation or percussion
Fecal impaction	Hard stool in vault, abdominal distension
Drugs/toxins	
Medications (eg, opioids, benzodiazepines, antihistamines)	
Drugs of abuse (eg, alcohol, methamphetamine, hallucinogens)	Miosis, mydriasis, anhidrosis
Withdrawals states (eg, alcohol, benzodiazepines)	Tachycardia, hypertension, labile blood pressure
Medication side effects (eg, serotonin syndrome, gabapentin toxicity, hyperammonemia)	Asterixis, myoclonus

(continued on next page)

Table 2
(continued)

Causes	Physical Examination Findings
Toxins (eg, ethylene glycol, methanol)	Depends on agent: salivation, lacrimation, anhidrosis, miosis
Infections	
Pneumonia	Bronchial breath sounds, crackles, egophony
Soft tissue (eg, cellulitis, pressure ulcer infection)	
Urinary tract infection	Suprapubic tenderness
Meningitis	Nuchal rigidity, Kernig and Brudzinski signs, positive jolt acceleration test

ascites, or jaundice, can provide evidence of possible hepatic encephalopathy. If able to follow commands, the patient should be assessed for the presence of asterixis. Although asterixis is often associated with hepatic encephalopathy, it is a nonspecific finding. Other common causes of asterixis include uremia, hypercarbia, drug side effects (most commonly antiepileptics), stroke, and viral encephalitis.[17] If asterixis is

Table 3
Causes of delirium in which examination characteristics exist

Cause	Physical Examination Findings	Sens	Spec	LR+	LR-
Meningitis[18]	Nuchal rigidity	46.1	71.3	1.60	0.76
	Kernig sign	22.9	91.2	2.61	0.84
	Brudzinski sign	27.5	88.8	2.44	0.82
	Jolt acceleration	52.4	71.1	1.81	0.67
Hypothyroidism[19]	Coarse skin	60.9	73.8	2.33	0.53
	Slow movements	87	13.1	1	1
	Bradycardia	43.5	88.8	3.88	0.64
	Pretibial edema	78.3	30.8	1.13	0.7
	Puffiness of face	91.3	20.6	1.15	0.42
	Delayed ankle reflex	47.8	86	3.41	0.61
	Coarse skin, bradycardia, ankle reflex	60	84	3.75	0.48
Hyperthyroidism[20]	Tachycardia (>90 beats/min)	80	82	4.5	0.2
	Skin moist and warm	34	95	6.8	0.7
	Enlarged thyroid	93	59	2.3	0.1
	Eyelid retraction	34	99	33.2	0.7
	Eyelid lag	19	99	18.6	0.8
	Fine finger tremor	69	94	11.5	0.3
Pneumonia[21]	Bronchial breath sounds	14–19	94–96	3.3	0.9
	Egophony	4–16	96–99	4.1	NS
	Crackles	19–67	36–97	2.8	0.8
	Diminished breath sounds	7–60	73–98	2.4	0.8
	Dullness to percussion	4–26	82–99	3.6	NS
	Asymmetric chest expansion	5	100	44.1	NS

Abbreviations: LR+, likelihood ratio positive; LR-, likelihood ratio negative, NS, not significant; Sens, sensitivity; Spec, specificity.

present, effort should be made to differentiate among these possibilities and avoid anchoring on hepatic encephalopathy.

Most of the physical examination findings for conditions causing delirium do not have robust data on test characteristics. **Table 3** lists potential causes of delirium for which there is some evidence in the literature supporting physical examination maneuvers. In addition, please refer to the articles in this issue "Chronic Obstructive Pulmonary Disease and the Physical Exam", "Cirrhosis" and "Congestive Heart Failure" on chronic obstructive pulmonary disease, cirrhosis, and congestive heart failure for evidence on those specific examinations.

For meningitis, physical examination maneuvers do not have very impactful LRs. The sensitivities are particularly low, so they are not very good at ruling out disease. In a study by Akaishi and colleagues a case was made for performing jolt accentuation (head rotation 2 to 3 times per second to see if headache worsens) in patients suspected as having meningitis over checking for nuchal rigidity because jolt accentuation is easier to reproduce, although both have comparable test characteristics.[18]

For hypothyroidism, the physical examination findings when considered in isolation also have poor diagnostic accuracy and test performance. However, the combination of coarse skin, bradycardia, and delayed ankle reflex taken together have modest diagnostic accuracy and might be useful to identify which patients should receive further laboratory testing in a search for underlying thyroid disease.[19]

The examination findings in hyperthyroidism are much more helpful to the clinician. The lack of a goiter or lack of tachycardia (heart rate >90) make this diagnosis much less likely (low LR−), whereas the presence of eyelid lag, eyelid retraction, or a fine tremor all have LR+ greater than 10, making the diagnosis much more likely.[20]

Last, the pulmonary examination for pneumonia has findings with modest LR+, such as crackles, egophony, and bronchial breath sounds.[21] Their presence on examination can be an important clue but are not diagnostic in most cases. Unfortunately, they are often absent in many patients with pneumonia, so their absence is not particularly helpful at ruling out pneumonia.

SUMMARY

Delirium is an acute and fluctuating disorder characterized by a disturbance in attention and cognition. Delirium is underdiagnosed by clinicians, but there are excellent diagnostic tools that use history and physical examination findings that can assist clinicians in making the diagnosis in multiple settings (ie, the CAM, CAM-ICU, 3d-CAM, b-CAM, 4AT, and UB-CAM). The UB-2 screen is a quick tool that can be used daily on all patients and that can reliably rule out delirium. If the screening result is positive, it can be followed with a more sensitive tool such as the 3D-CAM to confirm the diagnosis. Delirium is caused by underlying medical conditions and is often multifactorial, so a full diagnosis requires a careful assessment for a wide range of potential causes. Such an assessment includes a careful history, complete medication review, a thorough physical examination, and targeted laboratory and imaging studies. Other than the diagnostic tools discussed earlier, the physical examination for delirium has not been specifically studied. Though not specific to patients with delirium, some students show that some physical findings in meningitis, thyroid disease and pneumonia may have some value in daignosing these conditions, which may be causes of delirium. . Even without known test characteristics, a complete physical examination can provide potentially important clues to underlying conditions.

CLINICS CARE POINTS

- Delirium is an acute, fluctuating condition characterized by inattention and a change in cognition characterized by either disorganized thinking or a change in the level of consciousness.

- Delirium is one of the most common neuropsychiatric conditions affecting medical patients, especially those who are older and hospitalized.

- It is critical that delirium be recognized and addressed because it is often a clue to serious underlying medical conditions. However, delirium is not recognized by clinicians in 65% to 88% of cases.

- The CAM has been studied extensively and has the best test characteristics for diagnosing delirium in general medical patients. As it takes significant time to deliver, shorter, structured versions of this have been identified for the general medical (3D-CAM), ICU (ICU-CAM), and emergency department patients (bCAM) patients that have similar excellent test performance to diagnose delirium.

- For busy clinicians, the very quick, 2-item UB-2 screen in non-ICU patients is useful to rule out delirium if it is negative. Owing to its lower specificity, if the result of screening is positive it should be followed up by the 3D-CAM or 4AT diagnostic tool to confirm delirium.

- The history and physical examination provide important clues to the underlying cause for the delirium and may help determine whether laboratory tests and/or imaging are warranted.

- Common causes of delirium include medication side effects, infections, neurologic disorders, and metabolic disorders. However, clinicians should consider a broad differential in evaluating patients with delirium.

- There is limited evidence for test characteristics for physical examination findings associated with causes for delirium, but evidence does exist for diagnosing meningitis, cirrhosis, hypothyroidism, hyperthyroidism, and pneumonia.

DISCLOSURE

The authors have nothing to disclose.

REFERENCES

1. American Psychiatric Association. Neurocognitive disorders. In: Diagnostic and statistical manual of mental disorders. 5th edition. Arlington: American Psychiatric Publishing, Inc; 2013.
2. Wilson JE, Mart MF, Cunningham C, et al. Delirium. Nat Rev Dis Primers 2020;6:90.
3. Inouye SK, Westendorp RG, Saczynski JS. Delirium in elderly people. Lancet 2014;383:911–22.
4. Marcantonio ER. Delirium in hospitalized older adults. N Engl J Med 2017;377: 1456–66.
5. Wong CL, Holroyd-Leduc J, Simel DL, et al. Does this patient have delirium?: value of bedside instruments. JAMA 2010;304:779–86.
6. Inouye SK, van Dyck CH, Alessi CA, et al. Clarifying confusion: the confusion assessment method. Ann Intern Med 1990;113:941–8.
7. Inouye SK, Foreman MD, Mion LC. Nurses' recognition of delirium and its symptoms: comparison of nurse and researcher ratings. Arch Intern Med 2001;161: 2467–73.
8. Marcantonio ER, Ngo LH, O'Connor M, et al. 3D-CAM: derivation and validation of a 3- minute diagnostic interview for CAM-defined delirium. Ann Intern Med 2014; 161:554–61.

9. Ely EW, Margolin R, Francis J, et al. Evaluation of delirium in critically ill patients: validation of the confusion assessment method for the intensive care unit (CAM-ICU). Crit Care Med 2001;29:1370–9.
10. Ho M, Montgomery A, Traynor V, et al. Diagnostic performance of delirium assessment tools in critically ill patients: a systematic review and meta-analysis. Worldviews Evid Based Nurs 2020;17:301–10.
11. Han JH, Wilson A, Vasilevskis EE, et al. Diagnosing delirium in older emergency department patients: validity and reliability of the delirium triage screen and the brief confusion method. Ann Emerg Med 2013;62:457–65.
12. Bellelli G, Morandi A, Davis DH, et al. Validation of the 4AT, a new instrument for rapid delirium screening: a study in 234 hospitalised older patients. Age Ageing 2014;43:496–502.
13. Tieges Z, Maclullich AM, Anand A, et al. Diagnostic accuracy of the 4AT for delirium detection in older adults: systematic review and meta-analysis. Age Ageing 2021;50:733–43.
14. Fick DM, Inouye SK, Guess J, et al. Preliminary development of an ultrabrief two-item bedside test for delirium. J Hosp Med 2015;10:645–50.
15. Marcantonio ER, Fick DM, Jones RN, et al. The Ultra-brief confusion assessment method (UB-CAM): a new approach for rapid diagnosis of CAM-defined delirium. Network for Investigation of Delirium: Unifying Scientists; 2020. Available at: https://deliriumnetwork.org/the-ultra-brief-confusion-assessment-method-ub-cam/.
16. Moytl CM, Ngo L, Zhou W, et al. Comparative accuracy and efficiency of four delirium screening protocols. J Am Geriatr Soc 2020;68:2572–8.
17. Ellul MA, Cross TJ, Larner AJ. Asterixis. Pract Neurol 2017;17:60–2.
18. Aksaishi T, Kobayashi J, Abe M, et al. Sensitivity and specificity of meningeal signs in patients with meningitis. J Gen Fam Med 2019;20:193–8.
19. Indra R, Patil SS, Joshi R, et al. Accuracy of physical exam in the diagnosis of hypothyroidism: a cross-sectional, double blind study. J Postgrad Med 2004; 50:7–10.
20. McGee S. Thyroid and its disorders. In: Evidence-based physical diagnosis. 5th edition. Philadelphia: Elsevier; 2022. p. 208–12.
21. McGee S. Pneumonia. In: Evidence-based physical diagnosis. 5th edition. Philadelphia: Elsevier; 2022. p. 271–9.

Physical Examination in the Evaluation of Dementia

Ashleigh E.H. Wright, MD, Heather E. Harrell, MD

KEYWORDS

- Physical examination • Diagnosis • Dementia • Cognitive impairment

KEY POINTS

- Despite the benefits of early diagnosis, dementia is underdiagnosed worldwide.
- Physicians can screen for dementia in high-risk populations by using the Mini-Cog in combination with the Ascertain Dementia 8-Item Informant Questionnaire (AD8).
- Follow-up testing with the Montreal Cognitive Assessment (MoCA) or Mini-Mental State Examination (MMSE) can help to solidify a diagnosis of dementia.
- The physical examination in patients with suspected dementia is usually within normal limits, although some subtypes of dementia do have distinct physical examination findings.
- The physical examination is essential in the work-up of dementia, so that systemic diseases that can present with cognitive decline can be identified and treated appropriately.

INTRODUCTION
Nature of the Problem

Dementia is an extremely common, yet sometimes difficult to diagnose, medical concern. Globally, the prevalence of dementia is 5%.[1,2] Alzheimer type dementia affects 5% to 10% of people over age 65 years and up to 50% of those over 85 years of age.[3] For an average individual, the lifetime risk of dementia is about 17%.[2] In the United States, the prevalence of dementia is 15% in people older than 68 years.[3] In 2015, 46.8 million people carried a diagnosis of dementia worldwide, with numbers expected to double every 20 years until reaching 131.5 million in 2050.[1,3] Although the prevalence of dementia has slightly declined since 2000, the overall number of patients with dementia continues to rise as the number of older individuals in society increases.[2] With the increasing number of individuals diagnosed with dementia, specialists likely will not be able to keep up with the increased need for care, with much of the responsibility falling to primary care physicians.[1] Alzheimer's disease is the sixth leading cause of death and the fifth leading cause of death among people

University of Florida, PO Box 103204, 1329 SouthWest 16th Street, Suite 5140, Gainesville, FL 32610, USA
E-mail address: Ashleigh.Wright@medicine.ufl.edu

Med Clin N Am 106 (2022) 471–482
https://doi.org/10.1016/j.mcna.2021.12.009
0025-7125/22/© 2021 Elsevier Inc. All rights reserved.

older than 65 years.[3] Median survival time after a diagnosis of dementia from all causes is only 4.5 years.[2]

Medical costs associated with caring for individuals with dementia are significant. In 2015, the global sum of direct medical costs for dementia was estimated to be $818 billion, 1.1% of the global gross domestic product. By 2030, the global costs are estimated to rise to 2 trillion dollars.[1]

Despite the large numbers of people affected by dementia throughout the world, it is largely underdiagnosed. Approximately 61% of older people who meet the criteria for a diagnosis of dementia never receive any formal diagnosis of the condition.[4] In fact, only 19% of patients with a confirmed dementia diagnosis had been checked for dementia during routine medical care.[1]

Goals

Although there is no known cure for most common types of dementia, there are many benefits to establishing a diagnosis early. Early detection of a reversible cause of dementia maximizes the chance of reversing or at least stopping the progression of symptoms.[1] Furthermore, an accurate and specific diagnosis is necessary for targeting therapies to patients with these diagnoses.[1]

One of the most important reasons to establish a diagnosis of dementia is to allow individuals to plan their future medical care while they still have decisional capacity.[1] Without a formal diagnosis of dementia, access to elements of dementia management, such as medications, behavioral interventions, and caregiver support is unavailable.[1] As mortality risks overall for individuals with dementia are two times higher than those without dementia, anticipatory planning can be very important and time sensitive.[5]

Current Evidence

In 2014, the U.S. Preventive Services Task Force (USPSTF) found insufficient evidence to evaluate the balance of harms and benefits for universal screening for cognitive impairment with formal screening instruments in community dwelling adults age 65 years and over.[2,3] However, Alzheimer's Disease International, the International Association of Gerontologists and Geriatrics, and the Gerontological Society of America have encouraged active case finding among high-risk groups in ambulatory care settings.[4] Although some patients will report forgetfulness to their physician, others are unaware of a problem.[3] In fact, 20% of family informants failed to recognize memory problems in elderly patients who were found to have dementia on formal testing.[1] Screening at risk people for dementia in primary care practices significantly promotes the recognition of dementia.[1] Although age remains the greatest risk factor for the development of dementia, there are other risk factors, both modifiable and fixed.[6] Modifiable risk factors include hypertension, diabetes, poor diet, mid-life obesity, use of anticholinergic medications, and limited cognitive, physical, and social activities.[3] Fixed risk factors include family history of dementia, personal history of cardiovascular disease, personal history of cerebrovascular disease, apolipoprotein E4 genotype, and lower educational level.[3]

Dementia is described in the fifth edition of the Diagnostic and Statistical Manual of Mental Disorders (DSM-5) by the term "major neurocognitive disorder."[1,3] DSM-5 criteria for major neurocognitive disorders can be seen in **Fig. 1**.

It is necessary to clarify the diagnosis of dementia, as compared with the changes associated with normal aging and mild cognitive impairment (MCI).[7] The changes in memory and cognition seen with normal aging are mostly mild changes in memory and the rate of information processing. This should not interfere with daily

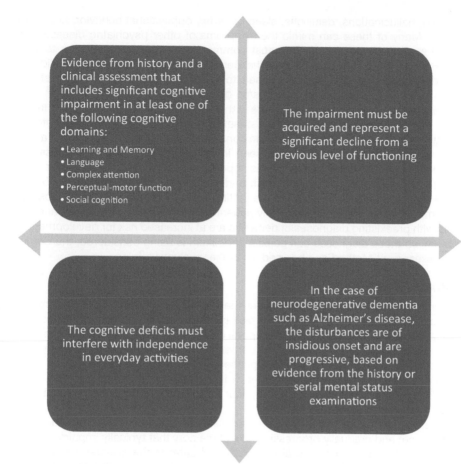

Fig. 1. DSM V criteria for diagnosis of major cognitive disorder.

functioning.[1] Although the ability to perform new learning or acquire new memories can decline with normal aging, cued recall should remain stable over time.[1]

Mild cognitive impairment is defined by the presence of memory difficulty and objective memory impairment, but with a preserved ability to function in daily life.[1,3] There is a measurable deficit in at least one of the 5 domains described in **Fig. 1**, identified by objective neurologic cognition tests.

Although there is no specific treatment of MCI, it is useful to make the diagnosis, as the annual conversion rate from MCI to dementia ranges from 6% to 25%. Not all of those with MCI will go on to develop dementia, and progression from normal memory to MCI to dementia is not always linear.[1]

Two other diagnoses that can present very similarly to dementia are depression and delirium. Major depression in the elderly can cause pseudodementia.[1] Depression can manifest with sadness, loss of interest, sleep disturbances, appetite changes, and feelings of worthlessness or guilt.[1] Dementia can sometimes coexist with depression, so it is important to assess for both when considering these diagnoses. Dementia can sometimes cause symptoms of disturbed perception, thought content, mood, and behavior.[1] More than half of the people with dementia will have behavioral and psychological symptoms. These symptoms can include verbal and physical aggression, agitation, hallucinations, delusions, sleep disorder, oppositional behavior, and wandering.[1] Many of these can mimic the symptoms of other psychiatric diseases, so careful evaluation is required. The most commonly used clinical screening tool for depression in an elderly population is the Geriatric Depression Scale. This validated tool, developed in 1982, was condensed to a brief 30-question self-administered test in 1986, and consists of entirely yes/no questions, lending to ease of use.[8]

Delirium is covered in depth elsewhere in this text, but should be considered in patients who have an acute or subacute onset in memory and cognition symptoms. Delirium is associated with fluctuations in consciousness, alteration in levels of attention and concentration, and is often seen in individuals with systemic illness.[1] In community-dwelling elderly patients, it is important to recall that delirium is relatively uncommon. A Canadian study of health and aging showed that less than 0.5% of elderly people outside of an acute care setting met the criteria for the diagnosis of delirium.[1] However, hospitalized elderly patients are more prone to delirium, and patients with preexisting diagnoses of dementia are at increased risk for development of delirium, so these diagnoses can coexist. If delirium is being considered, the Confusion Assessment Method can be used for further evaluation.[9]

Subtypes of Dementia

Dementia is an umbrella term that includes many distinct diseases. The most common subtypes of dementia are: Alzheimer's disease, followed by vascular dementia, dementia with Lewy bodies, and frontotemporal dementia.[5] These subtypes of dementia can occur in combination, with vascular dementia often being present to some extent. Less common subtypes can be misdiagnosed as Alzheimer's disease, but as some types of dementia have unique therapies, it is important to make an accurate diagnosis.[5] Elements of the history and physical examination can help differentiate between subtypes of dementia.

Alzheimer's disease affects executive and visuospatial function relatively early with a slow onset and gradually progressive loss of memory that typically impairs learning new, particularly autobiographical information.[1,3] Later in the disease, patients will develop a language deficit and behavioral symptoms.[1] A person with Alzheimer's disease will repeat questions and conversations.[3] Differentiating this condition from other causes of dementia is easiest in the early stage of illness, as dementia in its later stages has similar manifestations regardless of cause.[3]

Vascular dementia is caused by cerebrovascular disease and is divided into poststroke dementia and vascular dementia without recent stroke.[1] Thus, vascular dementia can share neurologic deficits seen in patients with poststroke, including sensory, motor, cerebellar, and other higher cortical deficits on the neurologic examination. Dementia with Lewy bodies can cooccur with symptoms of parkinsonism and has classic features of rapid eye movement (REM) sleep behavior disorder and fluctuation of cognition.[1] Frontotemporal dementia is early onset dementia with prominent changes of social behavior, personality, or aphasia.[1] Although less than 10% of total dementia diagnoses, frontotemporal dementia represents 60% of dementia cases in patients 45 to 60 years of age.[10]

DISCUSSION
Approach

No single test can confirm the diagnosis of dementia.[3] A thorough combination of history from the patient and caregiver, physical examination, cognitive assessment, laboratory evaluation, and neuroimaging must be used.[3] The history should detail the nature (domains impacted), magnitude (severity and impact on daily functioning), and course of cognitive changes (temporal course of symptoms, including speed of onset and pattern).[3,10] Early in the disease course, dementia often impairs instrumental activities of daily living, such as paying bills, balancing finances, or remembering medications.[3] The history taken in a patient with suspected dementia should also carefully rule out other possible causes of memory and cognitive complaints, through a review of family, medical, and psychiatric history.[3] This should specifically include a history of obstructive sleep apnea, cardiovascular disease, head trauma, alcohol use, and depression.[3] Medication review is essential.

The examination of a patient with possible dementia should begin with a general assessment. The patient's general appearance may offer clues to the possible cause and severity of cognitive complaints.[6] Patients with either dementia or depression may show signs of self-neglect or poor hygiene.[6]

Evaluation - Cognitive Testing

In 2013, the Alzheimer's Association recommended 3 dementia screening tests that could be completed during the Medicare wellness visit: the Mini-Cog, the Memory Impairment Screen, and the General Practitioner Assessment of Cognition.[2] The General Practitioner Assessment of Cognition incorporates a subjective and objective experience, but is only validated in Australian patient populations. After a meta-analysis brought into question, the sensitivity of the Memory Impairment Screen, the Ascertain Dementia 8-Item Informant Questionnaire (AD8) was introduced as a quick, validated, and sensitive screening tool.[2] The Alzheimer's Association currently advocates combining the Mini-Cog with the AD8 for in-clinic dementia screening.[2]

The Mini-Cog is a three-item recall and scored clock drawing test.[1] The Mini-Cog has many advantages. It is available for free at www.mini-cog.com. It has a high sensitivity for predicting dementia, is easily and quickly administered, and its diagnostic value is not limited by a patient's education or language. The Mini-Cog is administered by asking a patient to recall three words, with a score of 1, 2, or 3 based on the number of words recalled without cues. A patient also draws a clock which must include all numbers 1 to 12 in the correct order, with 2 hands pointing to the correct numbers. A total score of 3, 4, or 5 indicates lower likelihood of dementia, but does not rule out some degree of cognitive impairment.[1]

The AD8 dementia screening tool is an 8-item questionnaire whereby the patient and a close informant are asked to describe whether there are any changes in 8 deficits or behaviors.[1] A positive response to 2 or more questions has a sensitivity of 93% and specificity of 46% for dementia, making it an excellent component of a screening test, but necessitating follow-up with a more specific diagnostic tool.[1] The AD8 is available for free at https://www.alz.org/media/Documents/ad8-dementia-screening.pdf.

If a patient screens positive for dementia based on Mini-Cog and AD8 performance, then further testing is indicated. Two of the most commonly used tests are the Mini-Mental State Examination (MMSE) or Montreal Cognitive Assessment (MoCA). The MMSE is relatively brief, easy to administer, and is inclusive of multiple domains.[1] MMSE scores can be adjusted for patient age and education using a validated chart.[1] Also, the pattern of clinical deficit shown by the MMSE can be useful in the diagnosis of dementia.[1] However, the MMSE is not sensitive for the diagnosis of mild dementia, and has limited ability to assess cognitive decline over time.[1] Scores can be influenced by age, education, language, and motor/visual impairment, although as mentioned, some of this can be accounted for using available reference charts.[1] Importantly, the MMSE is copywritten, and therefore can only be used with a patient after purchase.

The MoCA is designed to detect cognitive impairment and is more sensitive overall than the MMSE for the detection of MCI. It includes a wider range of cognitive domains than the MMSE, and includes memory, language, attention, visuospatial skills, and executive function.[2] The MoCA is available free online, and there is also an abbreviated version, which only takes 5 minutes.[1] The major disadvantage is that the full version of the MoCA takes approximately 15 minutes to perform, significantly longer than the MMSE. **Table 1** provides a comparison of the main cognitive tests described above.

Comparisons of the AD8 screen alone, cognitive tests (e.g., MoCA or Mini-Cog) alone, and a combination of the AD8 with one of these tests showed that when the informant reports the AD8, it can be subject to recall and desirability bias, and therefore prone to diagnostic error. Cognitive tests are less prone to bias but can be more time-consuming and may require training. The Mini-Cog was 95% effective, and the MMSE was 92% effective in detecting dementia in one study.[4] In that same study, the MoCA was 85% effective and the MMSE was 76% effective in detecting MCI. Although all strategies for detecting dementia were effective, a combined measure had the best performance. Informant reports and brief cognitive tests, when used together, capture the 2 criteria that are needed for the definition of MCI and dementia—subjective reports of cognitive decline and objective evidence of cognitive deficits. For detecting MCI, only a combination of informant reporting and cognitive testing was statistically significant, as neither was sensitive enough to detect this subtler cognitive impairment alone.

Approach – Neurologic Examination

The physical examination can be extremely useful when evaluating suspected dementia. A comprehensive neurologic examination should be performed in all patients with cognitive decline. Although most forms of dementia will not have any associated findings, there are some typical findings seen in the most common forms of dementia. In addition to the findings mentioned in the previous section, vascular dementia, Lewy body dementia, and frontotemporal dementia all have some common findings seen on neurologic examination, including gait assessment.

As mentioned, in Alzheimer dementia, the physical examination will not necessarily provide any clues to the diagnosis, other than the lack of abnormal findings, which suggests primary dementia. Vascular dementia, the second most common cause of dementia, will often have findings consistent with areas of cerebral ischemia. Therefore, a complete neurologic examination is required for all patients with dementia. This includes a cranial nerve assessment, strength testing, reflex evaluation, sensory testing, and cerebellar and gait testing. Based on the size and location of ischemic lesions underlying the diagnosis of vascular dementia, there may or may not be abnormalities on the neurologic examination.

Frontotemporal dementia, as is suggested by its name, largely presents with frontal lobe deficits which manifest as abnormalities in executive function. These include trouble planning and organizing, apathy, and inappropriate behavior due to the lack of inhibition. Tremors, weakness, rigidity, and balance concerns may be present but are not required for diagnosis.[2]

Lewy body dementia and Parkinson's disease are clinical diagnoses with not only some similarities but also important differences. In Parkinson's disease, the examiner should look for a resting tremor, bradykinesia, rigidity, and loss of postural reflexes.[10] Lewy body dementia can be very difficult to diagnose, as the physical symptoms seen in parkinsonism are not expected early in the presentation. In Lewy body dementia, the dementia symptoms seem before or at the same time as any other parkinsonian features. Therefore, the practitioner should continually assess for the development

Table 1
Comparison of screening and diagnostic cognitive assessments

	Benefits	Drawbacks
Mini-Cog	Sensitive, easy to administer, not affected by education or language	Does not include all domains of cognitive impairment or subjective experience
General Practitioner Assessment of Cognition	Incorporates interview and objective testing, easy to use free website	Only validated in Australian populations
AD8	Brief, 8 question interview can be given to the patient and caregiver, and has high sensitivity	Low specificity, can be impacted by informant bias
MMSE	Sensitive for the diagnosis of moderate to advanced dementia, includes multiple domains of cognition	Impacted by personal demographics, not sensitive for mild dementia, copywritten
MoCA	Sensitive for detection of mild cognitive impairment, evaluates multiple cognitive domains, free online	Can take up to 15 minutes to perform

of these symptoms in follow-up visits. Often, there are no abnormal physical examination findings at the time of diagnosis of Lewy body dementia.

Approach – Gait Assessment

An in-depth evaluation of a patient's gait is essential in the diagnosis of dementia. Prevalence of gait disorders increases from 10% in people aged 60 to 69 years to more than 60% in community-dwelling adults aged over 80 years.[11] In two-thirds of patients with a gait disorder, the cause was neurologic, and among neurologic diagnoses, the most common causes are: sensory ataxia (18%), parkinsonian disorder (16%), and frontal brain disease (8%).[11] Studies have shown strong effects of cognition on gait, including the role of gait speed. Gait disorders that develop in older age can be an indicator for the future development of dementia.[11]

Cognitive control is relevant for avoiding obstacles and choosing the best walking route. Frontal executive function, special perception, and attention all contribute to walking; patients with dementia tend to walk more slowly due to a decline in these areas. However, patients with dementia also often walk too quickly in relation to the motor and cognitive deficits placing them at an increased risk of falls.[12]

Frontal gait disorder refers to a walking pattern that occurs in individuals who have forgotten how to perform the act of walking.[12] This is demonstrated by difficulty standing up, inadequately adopting new postures when changing position, and difficulty achieving a stable position. Patients with a frontal gait pattern also will have a broad-based gait with lateral arm extension with minimal arm swing. The trunk posture will frequently be abnormal, either stooped, upright, or hyper-extended.[12] This gait pattern can be seen in patients with vascular lesions, normal pressure hydrocephalus (NPH), advanced Alzheimer's disease, and frontotemporal dementia.

The parkinsonian gait is characterized by rigid, akinetic movement with slow gait, and short step length, narrow base, and stooped posture including the neck, shoulders, and trunk. These patients also will often have the other cardinal motor signs of Parkinson's disease, including bradykinesia, rigidity, rest tremor, and impaired postural stability. Even at very early stages of Lewy body dementia and Parkinson's disease, movement can seem somewhat slow. Asking the patient to perform other tasks while walking can worsen the parkinsonian gait.[12]

Patients with vascular dementia can have a wide variety of gait abnormalities based on whereby the cranial lesions are located. Focal neurologic deficits can affect motor and balance.

Focal neurologic signs or parkinsonism should be seen in the early stages of Lewy Body Disease (LBD).[3] Typical parkinsonian movement patterns include resting tremor, slowness, and gait imbalance.[12] These parkinsonian signs, upper motor neuron signs, or gait disturbances may indicate a potential underlying process, and guide further evaluation and testing.[6] Pathologic reflexes, such as the grasp, snout, glabellar, and palmomental reflex are frequently seen in more advanced dementia.[6]

Approach – Examination to Exclude Alternative Diagnoses

Although physical examination findings are typically normal in patients with dementia, they can assist in differential diagnosis generation.[2,6] Special attention should be given to the general assessment, skin examination, cardiovascular and pulmonary examinations, ENT and eye examination, and a thorough neurologic examination including gait evaluation. When noted, abnormalities in the physical examination can assist in finding potentially reversible causes of cognitive decline, including hypothyroidism, vitamin deficiency, neurosyphilis, tumors, normal-pressure hydrocephalus, depression, and hypoperfusion from heart failure.[2] A normal physical examination points toward a diagnosis of Alzheimer dementia. See **Table 2** for review.

Thyroid disease – Although no one single sign of hypothyroidism has an adequately large likelihood ratio to consistently differentiate a euthyroid from a hypothyroid patient, a combination of signs including coarse skin, bradycardia, and delayed ankle reflex have been shown to have modest accuracy (LR+ 3.75; LR- 0.48).[13]

Vitamin B12 deficiency – Vitamin B12 deficiency has a well-established association with memory loss, impaired cognition, and may coexist with dementia.[14] Repletion of B12 has been found to improve subjective memory, as well as MMSE scores, in most of the patients who were deficient.[15] B12 deficiency has many physical manifestations, which include skin hyperpigmentation and vitiligo, glossitis, hyporeflexia, and decreased proprioception and vibratory sense, which can in turn cause gait difficulties.[16]

Neurosyphilis – Neurologic involvement occurs in nearly 10% of patients with untreated syphilis, and should be considered in any patients with neurologic symptoms and a history of this infection. Vascular lesions from meningovascular syphilis and neuronal degeneration from parenchymatous syphilis are possible, which can manifest with the constellation of symptoms known as tabes dorsalis. These include ataxia, aphasia, paresis and sensory loss, hyperreflexia, visual changes, and hearing loss, along with cognitive changes.[17] A unique finding seen in neurosyphilis is the Argyll Robertson pupil, which is seen on physical examination as small, irregular pupils with light-near dissociation manifested by an absent light reflex but prompt constriction with near accommodation.[18]

Tumors – The presentation of a brain tumor will vary by its location, but can include: cognitive and personality changes, gait disturbances, aphasia, sensory or motor loss, visual field deficits, ataxia or dysmetria, and more.[19]

Table 2
Physical examination abnormalities seen in systemic diseases that may present with cognitive decline

Medical Diagnosis	Organ System Involved				
	Dermatologic	Cardiac	Pulmonary	Neurologic	ENT/eye
Hypothyroidism	Coarse skin	Bradycardia		Delayed ankle reflex	
B12 deficiency	Hyperpigmentation and vitiligo			Hyporeflexia, gait impairment, decreased proprioception and vibratory sense	Glossitis
Neurosyphilis				Ataxia, aphasia, paresis, sensory loss, hyperreflexia, visual changes, hearing loss, Argyll Robertson pupil	
Tumors				Unique neurologic exam findings based on location	
NPH				Impaired balance, unstable gait	
Heart failure		Third or fourth heart sound, JVD, and peripheral edema	Rales and decreased breath sounds at bases		
Hepatolenticular degeneration (Wilson disease)					Kayser Fleischer rings

Normal pressure hydrocephalus (NPH) – The patient with NPH will demonstrate abnormalities in balance, gait, and cognitive functions. The remainder of the physical examination is expected to be normal. The gait abnormality in NPH is best described as a magnetic gait, whereby a person's feet seem to be attached to the floor as if by a magnet. The impairment should be symmetric.[20] NPH has a unique historical feature in that urinary urgency and incontinence become prominent relatively early in the disease course.

Heart failure – To assist in making a diagnosis of heart failure, the physician should evaluate for jugular venous distention and peripheral edema on the vascular examination, a displaced apical impulse and third or fourth heart sound on cardiac examination, and crackles or decreased breath sounds at the bases on pulmonary examination, as these are all findings that can be seen in isolation or in combination in the presence of heart failure.[21] A cardiovascular examination should thus be performed on any patient with cognitive decline to assure that heart failure and subsequent hypoperfusion of the brain is not a contributor.

Genetic diseases – The breadth of genetic diseases that can cause cognitive changes is beyond the scope of this article. However, one of the more common of these genetic disorders to consider is hepatolenticular degeneration (Wilson disease), a copper storage disorder. Ophthalmologic examination should be performed in all patients with cognitive decline or behavioral changes and can provide clues to conditions such as Wilson's disease, which may present with golden brown eye discoloration from Kayser Fleischer rings, best seen on slit-lamp examination.[3]

Recommendations

Fig. 2 simplifies the workflow for evaluating a patient with subjective memory concerns. When a patient presents to clinic, a physician should perform screening with the Mini-Cog and AD8. If a patient screens positive with this combination of evaluations, then the physician should test further with the MoCA or MMSE. If the initial testing is negative, the patient should still be evaluated for MCI (which is not easily detected on these tests) and monitored for progression to dementia in later years.

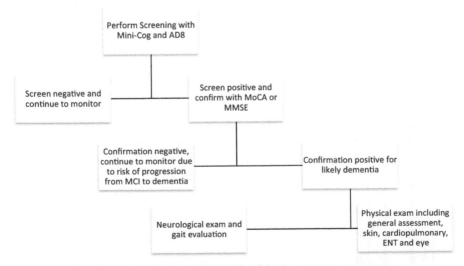

Fig. 2. Workflow for evaluating a patient with subjective memory concerns.

Based on clinician suspicion, neuropsychological testing could be performed to detect more subtle changes in memory, such as MCI.[7] If the MoCA or MMSE is positive, then the patient should have a thorough examination as detailed in this article, with the goals of diagnosing and treating possible contributing systemic diseases, and further refining the likely type of dementia from which the patient is suffering. A referral to a neurologist specializing in cognitive concerns is appropriate after a diagnosis of dementia is suspected, although as described in the introduction to this article, access to specialists is not keeping up with demand.

Future Directions – Prediction of Dementia based on Physical Examination

The physical examination can be used not only to assist in the diagnosis of dementia but also to predict the development of dementia in later years. The 2 most significant physical examination abnormalities that can predict the development of dementia within the next 10 years are difficulties with hand strength grip and single-leg balancing. Poor performance on hand strength grip testing or single leg balancing could be related to frailty or sedentary lifestyle, which is known to be a risk factor for dementia.[5] However, simply using the FRAIL scale to identify patients with a high subjective degree of frailty (fatigue, resistance, ambulation, illness, and loss of weight) was not predictive of incident dementia.[6] Other tests currently used to assess dementia (specifically MMSE and the clock drawing test) are not predictive of 10-year development of dementia.[5] It is not known if efforts to improve strength could decrease the likelihood of dementia development over the following 10 years for patients found to have abnormalities in grip strength or balance.[5]

CLINICS CARE POINTS

- Physicians should carefully screen at-risk patients for possible dementia, as symptoms of this important diagnosis are frequently under-reported by both patients and family members.
- Screening can be performed quickly and with high sensitivity through a combination of the Mini-Cog and AD8 questionnaire.
- Follow-up of a positive dementia screening test should be done with either a MoCA or MMSE.
- Patients who screen negative for dementia should be followed up regularly, as patients with subjective complaints of cognitive concerns have a higher risk of developing dementia in the future.
- Physical examination in the evaluation of dementia should include a general assessment, skin, cardiopulmonary, ENT, eye, and thorough neurologic evaluation.
- Goals of the physical examination in the assessment of dementia include diagnosing possible contributing systemic illnesses and also identifying the possible subtype of dementia occurring in a patient.
- Physicians should become proficient in making a diagnosis of dementia, as this disease is increasing in frequency as the numbers of patients over age 65 continues to increase.

ACKNOWLEDGMENTS

Thank you very much to Dr Heather Harrell for her wonderful mentorship, and for providing helpful feedback on this article.

DISCLOSURE

The author has nothing to disclose.

REFERENCES

1. Lam K, Chan WSY, Luk JKH, et al. Assessment and diagnosis of dementia: a review for primary healthcare professionals. Hong Kong Med J 2019;25(6):473–82.
2. Falk N, Cole A. Evaluation of Suspected Dementia. Am Fam Physician 2018; 97(6):398–405.
3. Arvanitakis Z, Shah RC, Bennett DA. Diagnosis and management of dementia: review. JAMA 2019;322(16):1589–99.
4. Liew TM. Active case finding of dementia in ambulatory care settings: a comparison of three strategies. Eur J Neurol 2020;27(10):1867–78.
5. Dallora AL, Minku L, Mendes E, et al. Multifactorial 10-year prior diagnosis prediction model of dementia. Int J Environ Res Public Health 2020;17(18):6674.
6. Hildreth KL, Church S. Evaluation and management of the elderly patient presenting with cognitive complaints. Med Clin North Am 2015;99(2):311–35.
7. Nelson AP, O'Connor MG. Mild cognitive impairment: a neuropsychological perspective. CNS Spectr 2008;13(1):56–64.
8. Aikman GG, Oehlert ME. Geriatric depression scale: long form versus short form. Clin Gerontol 2001;22(3–4):63–70.
9. Inouye S, van Dyck C, Alessi C, et al. Clarifying confusion: The confusion assessment method. Ann Intern Med 1990;113(12):941–8.
10. Jankovic J. Parkinson's disease: clinical features and diagnosis. J Neurol Neurosurg Psychiatr 2008;79(4):368–76.
11. Pirker W, Katzenschlager R. Gait disorders in adults and the elderly: A clinical guide. Wien Wien Klin Wochenschr 2017;129(3–4):81–95. https://doi.org/10.1007/s00508-016-1096-4.
12. Nicastri C, Hensley J, Lane S. Managing the Forgetful Patient: Best Practice for Cognitive Impairment. Med Clin North Am 2021;105(1):75–91.
13. Indra R, Patill SS, Joshi R, et al. Accuracy of physical examination in the diagnosis of hypothyroidism: a cross-sectional, double-blind study. J Postgrad Med 2004;50(1):7–11.
14. Jensen GL, Binkley J. Clinical manifestations of nutrient deficiency. JPEN J Parenter Enteral Nutr 2002;26(5 Suppl):S29–33.
15. Jatoi Shazia, Hafeez Abdul, Urooj Riaz Syeda, et al. Low Vitamin B12 Levels: An Underestimated Cause Of Minimal Cognitive Impairment And Dementia. Cureus 2020;12(2):e6976.
16. Langan R, Goodbred A. Vitamin B12 deficiency: recognition and management. Am Fam Physician 2017;96(6):384–9.
17. Brown D, Frank J. Diagnosis and management of syphilis. Am Fam Physician 2003;68(2):283–90.
18. Thompson HS, Kardon RH. The argyll robertson pupil. J Neuroophthalmol 2006; 26(2):134–8.
19. Perkins A, Liu G. Primary brain tumors in adults: diagnosis and treatment. Am Fam Physician 2016;93(3):211–217B.
20. Williams MA, Malm J. Diagnosis and treatment of idiopathic normal pressure hydrocephalus. continuum (Minneap Minn) 2016;22(2 Dementia):579–99.
21. Shamsham F, Mitchell J. Essentials of the Diagnosis of heart failure. Am Fam Physician 2000;61(5):1319–28.

Diabetes Physical Examination

Aamir Malik, MBBS[a], Sonia Ananthakrishnan, MD[b],*

KEYWORDS

- Diabetes mellitus • Diabetic examination • Blood pressure in diabetes
- Diabetic retinopathy • Diabetic peripheral neuropathy • Insertion site infections

KEY POINTS

- Physical examination of a patient with diabetes helps to identify both hallmark features linked to diabetes and key findings associated with the complications of diabetes.
- Blood pressure assessment is a key part of the physical exam of patients with diabetes to assist in evaluating risk of both micro- and macrovascular complications
- Assessment for diabetic retinopathy by a trained specialist is a vital part of the routine physical exam for patients with diabetes to identify individuals at risk for eventual vision loss
- Assessment for signs of peripheral neuropathy on physical exam is a key step to help prevent diabetic foot ulcers.

INTRODUCTION

Diabetes mellitus (DM) is characterized by hyperglycemia due to (a) inadequate production of insulin, most classically associated with type 1 insulin-dependent DM and/or (b) progressive insulin resistance, resulting in relative insulin deficiency, as seen in type 2 DM. With the overall prevalence of diabetes among adults in the United States estimated to range from 10.5% to 21.4% percent, this condition accounts for the utilization of more health care resources than any other health condition.[1,2] While polyuria and polydipsia are the hallmark symptoms of these conditions, most of the patients presenting with diabetes are asymptomatic, with hyperglycemia detected on routine or screening laboratory evaluation, prompting further assessment.

This underlies the importance of physical examination in patients with diabetes. Although early in the course of the disease the physical examination of a patient

[a] Diabetes and Nutrition, Boston University School of Medicine/Boston Medical Center, Section of Endocrinology, Diabetes and Nutrition, 720 Harrison Avenue, DOB 8th Floor, Boston, MA 02118; [b] Boston University School of Medicine/Boston Medical Center, Section of Endocrinology, Diabetes and Nutrition, 72 East Concord Street, Evans 122, Boston, MA, 02118
* Corresponding author:
E-mail address: Soniaa@bu.edu
Twitter: @SoniaAnan8 (S.A.)

Med Clin N Am 106 (2022) 483–494
https://doi.org/10.1016/j.mcna.2021.12.007
0025-7125/22/© 2022 Elsevier Inc. All rights reserved.

with diabetes may be unrevealing, there is an ongoing risk of end-organ damage increasing with the duration of diabetes. Physical examination plays an important role in recognizing hallmark features linked to diabetes and identifying key features associated with the complications of diabetes. The discussion of elements of the physical examination that can be performed by providers who are engaging in the patient-centered medical care of patients with diabetes will be reviewed in this article.

DISCUSSION
Assessment of Vital Signs

Blood pressure and pulse

Vitals signs are a critical starting point in a physical examination for a patient with diabetes. Measuring blood pressure at each visit and identifying the presence of hypertension in patients with diabetes can detect those at an increased risk of both macrovascular and microvascular disease, for example, cardiovascular or kidney disease.[3] Instituting early and effective treatment of hypertension in such patients can start to reduce the cardiovascular risk and preserve renal function.

Blood pressure assessment for patients with diabetes should occur at every routine clinical visit by a trained health care provider. Blood pressure should be measured after 5 minutes of rest, while the patient is in the seated position, with their feet on the floor and the arm supported at heart level. Appropriate cuff size should be selected based on the upper-arm circumference. Additional modalities such as home blood pressure self-monitoring and 24-h ambulatory blood pressure monitoring may assist in diagnosing white coat hypertension or other inconsistencies between blood pressure measurements on physical examination in the clinical setting and the patient's actual blood pressure.

Patients identified as having elevated blood pressure readings should have repeat measurements performed to confirm the presence of hypertension.[4] Hypertension affects approximately ~20% to 60% of patients with diabetes, depending on other factors such as obesity, ethnicity, and age.[5] Within the general population, stage 1 hypertension is defined as a blood pressure 130 to 139/80 to 89 mm Hg and stage 2 hypertension is ≥ 140/90 mm Hg.[6] The American Association of Clinical Endocrinologists recommends screening for diabetes in asymptomatic individuals who have a diagnosis of hypertension.[7]

For patients with diabetes, target blood pressure goals can be individualized, incorporating patient risk, side effects of anti-hypertensive medications, and patient preference.[8] In alignment with the 2017 American College of Cardiology/American Heart Association (ACC/AHA) guidelines on hypertension and updated in the Standards of Medical Care in Diabetes by the American Diabetes Association (ADA), intensive blood pressure control may be desired for patients with diabetes and existing atherosclerotic cardiovascular disease (ASCVD) or 10-year ASCVD risk of equal or greater than 15%.[6,9] In this population, it may be reasonable to target a pressure of less than 130/80 mm Hg if it can be safely attained. For patients with diabetes and hypertension at a lower 10-year ASCVD risk (less than 15%), the blood pressure goal is well-established to be less than 140/90. Measurement of blood pressure should be a part of every clinical encounter to identify those at risk and assist patients in achieving desired targets.

In addition to identifying patients with hypertension and the related cardiovascular risk, patients with established diabetes who are developing autonomic neuropathy may have postural changes in blood pressure. Simultaneous measurement of the pulse (reported as beats per minute) with blood pressure is an important part of assessing patient with diabetes, given that relative tachycardia is a typical finding in autonomic neuropathy often preceding the development of orthostatic hypotension.

Orthostatic hypotension is defined as a fall in the blood pressure of greater than 20/10 mm Hg after standing for 3 minutes. Assessment for orthostatic hypotension should occur at the initial visit with a patient with diabetes, and subsequently as indicated to detect autonomic dysfunction. Autonomic dysfunction is a long-term, debilitating complication of diabetes and is typically irreversible as well as difficult to manage medically. Orthostatic vital signs additionally may be useful in assessing volume status in patients with diabetes, particularly if hyperglycemia has contributed to volume loss through osmotic diuresis.

Height, weight, and body mass index

As the prevalence of diabetes—specifically, type 2 DM—is expected to double by the year 2030, the prevalence of excess body weight is similarly increasing.[2] The prevalence of obesity and severe obesity is anticipated to rise by 33% and 130%, respectively, in the next 2 decades.[10] Excess body weight and a sedentary lifestyle are associated with an increased risk of developing various diseases, particularly type 2 DM. Assessment of body weight is a key component to identifying patients to screen for diabetes as well as assessing risk and managing the health of patients with diabetes.[7]

Body mass index (BMI) for which weight in kilograms is divided by height in meters, expressed as kg/m2, is the World Health Organization (WHO) recommended index of weight-for-height. BMI can assist in classifying obesity in adults as well as assessing the risk for diabetes in all ethnic groups. Even modest weight gain is associated with an increased risk of type 2 DM and conversely, weight loss is associated with a reduced risk of type 2 DM.[11,12]

Additional data can be obtained by the assessment of waist circumference, as abdominal obesity provides independent diabetic risk information not captured by the BMI. The waist circumference is measured with a flexible tape starting at the horizontal plane of the iliac crest as seen from the anterior view.

Funduscopic Examination

The ophthalmologic examination is a key element of the physical examination of patients with diabetes. A diagnostic imperative in patients with diabetes is diabetic retinopathy (DR), a leading cause of blindness in the US. The duration that a patient has had diabetes, glycemic control achieved during the course of the disease as well as other risks such as hypertension, hyperlipidemia, and the presence of other microvascular complications such as nephropathy and/or neuropathy all help determine a patient's risk of developing retinopathy.[13]

Most of the patients who are developing DR will not experience symptoms until late in the disease process when macular edema or proliferative retinopathy has already occurred. At this point in disease evolution, therapy may be less effective. This highlights the importance of performing an initial screening examination for patients early, at the time of diagnosis of diabetes for patients with type 2 DM and within 5 years of diagnosis for patients with type 1 DM.

Routine screening should be repeated on an individualized basis, at least every 1 to 2 years in patients with well-controlled glycemia, with a dilated fundus examination or retinal photography to identify the development of retinal disease.[13] Typically, this assessment is conducted by providers with expertise, including ophthalmologists, optometrists or trained photographers working in conjunction with a skilled reader for the retinal photography. If prior examinations have not revealed any retinopathy, the subsequent assessment can occur with a retinal photographer and reader.[14]

Digital stereoscopic retinal imaging is now increasingly available in areas whereby access to specialty care may be limited, thus improving efficiency and reducing the cost of the examination for retinopathy. This technology uses a computer algorithm for evaluation, takes 15 to 20 minutes, does not require dilation of the eyes, and can be performed in a primary care provider's office with an ophthalmologist reading images remotely. In comparing the 3-image digital imaging with the gold standard 7-field stereoscopic fundus photography for retinopathy screening, both had similar sensitivity and specificity for detecting retinopathy.[15]

In routine office assessments, the eye examination should include a careful view of the retina, with the visualization of the optic disc and the macula. If hemorrhages or exudates are seen, this may serve as another prompt for the provider to refer to an ophthalmologist as soon as possible, to identify stages of progression of retinopathy. Examiners who are not ophthalmologists may underestimate the severity of retinopathy on the examination, especially if the patients' pupils are not dilated, again highlighting the need for specialist care to identify this common microvascular complication that carries a large burden.[16]

Oral Examination

There is growing evidence that oral health and the presence of periodontal disease are correlated with diabetes risk. This relationship may have multiple associations. Patients with diabetes have been noted to have improved glycemic control when treated for existing periodontal disease.[17] In addition, poorly controlled diabetes may be a marker for risk of severe periodontitis as well as poor response to periodontal treatments.[18]

These complex associations highlight the need for an oral examination to be part of the routine assessment of a patient with diabetes. Primary care providers may notice early signs of the development of both periodontitis and gingivitis with a simple oral inspection that reveals bad breath, gum swelling, and bleeding. These findings may trigger the provider to refer the patient to a dental professional for further evaluation and management.

Thyroid Examination

As per the ADA's Standards of Medical Care in Diabetes 2020 annual update, patients with type 1 DM should be screened for autoimmune thyroid disease on the diagnosis of diabetes.[4] They should be longitudinally re-assessed for thyroid disease annually.

This screening and follow-up assessment can include the palpation of the thyroid to detect diffuse enlargement involving the thyroid isthmus and lateral lobes. Enlargement could be suggestive of a goiter which can be found in either Hashimoto's thyroiditis, the most common form of autoimmune thyroid disease, as well as Grave's disease, an autoimmune cause of hyperthyroidism. However, it is important to note that a normal thyroid on palpation does not rule out the autoimmune thyroid disease that may be associated with type 1 DM. In cases whereby autoimmunity is being assessed, the thyroid physical examination should be followed up with biochemical assessment for autoimmune thyroid disease, most notably including a serum thyroid-stimulating hormone (TSH) level and antibodies against thyroid peroxidase (anti-TPO), an enzyme normally found in thyroid glands that plays an important role in the production of thyroid hormones.

Cardiovascular Examination

A comprehensive cardiovascular physical examination is not part of the Standards of Medical Care in Diabetes as recommended by the ADA.[4] However, elements of the cardiovascular examination may be important to identify specific cardiovascular complications. These may include assessing for findings consistent with ASCVD, including coronary heart disease, cerebrovascular disease, or peripheral artery disease (PAD). In addition, physical examination findings consistent with heart failure may be relevant in a patient with diabetes, whereby rates of heart failure hospitalizations are twice as high compared with patients without diabetes.[8] On physical examination, findings of tachycardia, irregular heart rate, S3 or S4, heart murmurs (eg, mitral regurgitation or ventricular septal defect), high or low blood pressure, lower extremity edema, and an elevated jugular venous pressure may be associated with these cardiovascular conditions.

Assessment of pulses as part of a thorough vascular examination may be relevant for patients with diabetes who have historical findings suggestive of PAD. A history of claudication, impaired walking function, and atypical non–joint-related lower extremity symptoms may prompt further examination. Physical examination findings suggestive of PAD include abnormal pulses, audible bruits, nonhealing lower extremity wounds, delayed capillary refill, cool extremities, and the presence of lower extremity gangrene. Patients with one or more of these findings should undergo ankle-brachial index (ABI) testing to further screen for PAD. See also *"Comprehensive Diabetic Foot Examination"* later in discussion.

For all patients with diabetes, routine assessment of cardiovascular risk criteria is a critical component to identifying patients who may benefit from more intensive risk factor management.[8] Cardiovascular risk factor assessment includes blood pressure examination (described above), as well as evaluating for historical and biochemical factors such as personal smoking history and fasting lipid profile.

Comprehensive Diabetic Foot Examination

Elliott Joslin mentioned in 1934 "diabetic gangrene is not heaven-sent, but earthborn."[19] For patients with type 1 or type 2 DM, the lifetime risk of a foot ulcer can be as high as 34%.[20] These preventable events are associated with a 2.5-fold risk of death compared with patients with diabetes without foot ulcers.[21] Patients with other complications including DR and nephropathy, especially those on dialysis, are at an increased risk for foot ulcers.[22]

On physical examination, a key step for practitioners is to begin with the patient removing their shoes and socks to examine the feet for the presence of callus, deformity, muscle wasting, and dry skin, all of which are clearly visible on inspection. A systematic approach to evaluate the feet of a patient with diabetes includes a history to direct the examination, dermatologic general inspection, and musculoskeletal, neurologic, and vascular assessments.

A basic history that may guide the foot examination includes assessment for prior foot ulceration or amputation and foot and leg discomfort, including numbness, tingling, claudication, and rest pain. Other factors that may impact foot care can include impaired vision, dialysis dependency, and tobacco use.[23]

A dermatologic assessment can include a global inspection for the presence of ulceration or areas of abnormal erythema, including within interdigital spaces. An assessment for appropriate nail care may reveal onychomycosis, which presents with findings of discoloration, subungual hyperkeratosis, splitting, and nail plate destruction. Also commonly seen in patients with diabetes may be tinea pedis, representing a fungal dermatophyte infection of the epidermis of the foot, with erosions or scales between the toes, and hyperkeratosis on the soles, medial and lateral surfaces of the feet, in a "moccasin" distribution. Other findings of callus (in particular with hemorrhage), nail dystrophy, paronychia, and focal or global skin temperature differences between feet may also prompt referral to a specialist.

On examination, the foot musculoskeletal assessment should include evaluation for any gross deformity. Rigid deformities may be found in the digits, causing contractures. Common forefoot deformities such as claw toe, which is metatarsal phalangeal joint hyperextension with interphalangeal flexion, and hammer toe, a distal phalangeal extension, can increase plantar pressures that cause skin breakdown. Charcot arthropathy, presenting as a unilateral, red, hot, swollen, flat foot with profound deformity is often misdiagnosed and may require immediate attention with referral to a podiatrist.

Peripheral neuropathy is the most common finding in the pathway to diabetic foot ulceration, seen in 80% of cases, highlighting the importance of the neurologic assessment of the feet.[13] This assessment can include 5 simple clinical tests including the 10 g monofilament, 128 Hz tuning fork, pinprick sensation, ankle reflexes and vibration perception threshold testing (**Table 1**). Ideally, 2 of the 5 tests should be regularly performed during the routine screening examinations, most commonly the 10 g monofilament with one other test. One or more abnormal tests suggest the loss of protective sensation. The inability to perceive pressure from a 10 g monofilament and a vibrating 128 Hz tuning fork over the hallux, and absent ankle reflexes all have been shown to be strong predictors of foot ulceration.[13,24]

Sensory neuropathy in combination with clinical evidence of PAD is another powerful predictor of future foot ulcers, highlighting the importance of the vascular examination of the feet. This examination can include the palpation of the presence of posterior tibial and dorsalis pedis pulses. Patients with diabetes with signs or symptoms of vascular disease or absent pulses on screening foot examination should undergo ABI testing and be considered for referral to a vascular specialist.

All patients with diabetes must have their feet evaluated yearly for the presence of neuropathy, vascular disease, and deformities. Once detected, a comprehensive foot

Table 1
Tests to detect peripheral neuropathy as part of the comprehensive diabetic foot examination

Test	Neurologic Impairment	Examination Notes
10 g monofilament	Protective sensation and large-fiber function	10 g monofilament is used to evaluate sensation at 12 sites which represent the most common areas of ulcer formation. Failure to detect cutaneous pressure at any site indicates a high risk for future ulceration
128 Hz tuning fork	Protective sensation and large-fiber function	Tuning fork is applied to the bony prominence at the dorsum of the first toe. Patient reports the perception of the start of vibration and cessation of vibration on dampening
Vibration perception threshold testing	Protective sensation and large-fiber function	Biothesiometer (electronic tuning fork) is placed on the pulp of big toe to detect the lowest voltage at which vibration can be sensed
Pinprick sensation	Protective sensation and small-fiber function	New, clean safety pin is used to test foot sensation. Pin should be discarded in a sharps container after use
Ankle reflexes	Both sensory and motor function	Reflex hammer is used to elicit reflex on Achilles tendons bilaterally while foot is dorsiflexed

examination may be performed at each routine clinical visit. It is through systematic examination, risk assessment, patient education, and timely referral to podiatry and/or vascular medicine that the high prevalence of lower extremity morbidity can be reduced.

SKIN EXAMINATION

According to various studies, 30% to 91% of patients with diabetes experience at least one dermatologic complication.[25,26] Given that diabetic conditions are so common, this highlights the importance of a skin examination that should include both inspection in specific anatomic regions as well as descriptions of specific skin findings. The discussion that follows describes specific findings on the skin physical examination relevant to patients with diabetes. Cutaneous manifestations of diabetes include common skin conditions and other findings such as insertion site complications and infections.

Common Skin Conditions

Acanthosis nigricans is a common disorder characterized by hyperchromic, velvety plaques located in intertriginous areas such as the axillae, groin, and posterior neck. It is usually asymptomatic, but may be painful, malodorous, or macerated in rare cases. There are 2 forms of acanthosis nigricans, benign and malignant, which share a similar clinical and histologic presentation. Benign acanthosis nigricans characteristically occurs in the setting of type 2 DM and obesity. It is also associated with other endocrine abnormalities involving insulin resistance and adjacent to diabetes including polycystic ovarian syndrome, lipodystrophy, acromegaly, and Cushing's syndrome. (See Kristen D. Kelley and Paul Aronowitz ' article ,"Disease-Based Physical Examination ," in this issue.)

Diabetic dermopathy, also called shin spots or pigmented pretibial patches, occurs in approximately one-half of patients with diabetes, most often in patients with microangiopathic complications.[27,28] Examination findings include multiple asymptomatic, round, dull red to pink papules or plaques predominantly located on the pretibial skin. Lesions evolve in one to 2 weeks to well-circumscribed, atrophic, brown macules and patches, often with a fine scale.

Skin tags are benign, asymptomatic, exophytic growths that can be found on the eyelids, neck, axilla, and other skin folds. They may be flesh-colored or, less often, hyperpigmented, and can range from small papules to pedunculated polyps, typically 1 to 6 mm in diameter, with smooth or irregular surfaces.

Vitiligo is an asymptomatic, acquired, chronic, depigmenting disorder of the skin characterized by achromic macules of selectively destroyed melanocytes. On examination, areas of depigmented skin can be found anywhere on the body with a preference for the face, areas around the orifices, genitals, and hands. They can vary in size from a few millimeters to many centimeters and usually have well-demarcated convex borders. It has been observed that patients with type 1 diabetes are significantly more likely to have vitiligo compared with those with type 2 diabetes (3.6% vs 0.4%).[29,30] There may also be a higher incidence in patients with type 2 diabetes compared with the general population.[31,32]

Psoriasis is a relatively common, chronic inflammatory skin disease with systemic manifestations. Physical examination will reveal red, itchy scaly patches most commonly on the knees, elbows, trunk, and scalp. Patients with psoriasis are believed to have 1.5 times increased risk of developing diabetes compared with the general population and patients with severe psoriasis may have twice that risk.[33]

Others Skin Findings

Insulin and insertion site skin reactions

The alterations of fat occurring at the insulin injection sites can create a small dimple or crater, known as lipodystrophy. This uneven fat distribution can lead to inadequate insulin absorption and poor glycemic control for those using insulin through subcutaneous injections or a pump.

With the advent of continuous glucose monitoring sensors and insulin pumps, it is not uncommon to encounter allergic skin reactions, lipodystrophy (as mentioned above), and skin infections. These occur at device insertions sites including the upper arm, forearm, abdomen, upper buttocks, upper hip (flank), and upper thigh (inner and outer areas). They present as hives, eczema, reddening of the skin, and uneven fat distribution.

Dermatologic complications are often a barrier for device use and an eventual reason for device discontinuation. Strategies to prevent skin complications include the identification of multiple sites for device insertion to allow insertion site rotation, use of medical-grade adhesives, good skin care, careful removal techniques, and adequate time for healing before new placement. Diabetes educators, providers, and patients all play an important role in examining the skin insertion sites and improving skin care for patients using devices in the management of diabetes. Partnering with patients using devices in this manner can increase the likelihood of success and satisfaction with device use.

Skin infections: fungal

Recurrent fungal infections such as tinea corporis and onychomycosis can be a presenting sign of diabetes. Tinea corporis appears as a ring-shaped patch or plaque which begins as a pruritic, circular, oval, erythematous, or hyperpigmented, scaling lesion that spreads centrifugally. Later, there is central clearing while a raised border remains. It appears on body sites other than the feet, groin, face, or hand. Onychomycosis, a common nail fungal infection, and tinea pedis are described elsewhere in this article (see the section on Comprehensive Diabetic Foot Examination).

Skin infections: bacterial

The most common bacterial skin infections in patients with diabetes are staphylococcal and beta-hemolytic streptococcal infections. Bacterial infections of the diabetic skin can range from mild infections to severe manifestations such as gangrene and even necrotizing fasciitis. Gangrene, as commonly found in diabetic foot infections, can be either dry or wet. Dry gangrene is manifested by a hard and dry skin texture with a clear demarcation between healthy and necrotic tissue, often affecting the distal aspects of toes and fingers. Wet gangrene seems as moist, gross swelling with blistering, and is a surgical emergency.

A diagnostic imperative, necrotizing fasciitis can manifest as erythema, edema, severe pain which is out of proportion to examination, crepitus, skin bullae, necrosis, or ecchymosis. Systemic features of fever, tachycardia, and hypotension may be present. Identifying the margins between necrotic tissue and healthy, viable, bleeding tissue is critical as this condition is a surgical emergency and the goal is to perform aggressive debridement of all necrotic tissue.

Psychosocial Examination

Paramount to patients achieving the treatment targets for diabetes is the maintenance of psychological well-being. To support this, providers can include psychosocial care into their collaborative, patient-centered medical care.[34] This can include a routine

Table 2
Significant components of the diabetes physical examination and frequency of examination related to patients with type 1 and type 2 DM

Physical Examination Component	Type 1 DM	Type 2 DM
Vital Signs: Blood pressure measurement	Every visit	Every visit
Vital Signs: Height, Weight, and BMI	Every visit	Every visit
Fundoscopic examination, with referral to specialty care	Within 5 y of diagnosis, and then at least every 1–2 y, with individualized frequency	At diagnosis, and then at least every 1–2 y, with individualized frequency
Thyroid examination	At diagnosis, and then annually	Annually
Foot examination	Within 5 y of diagnosis and then annually, or every visit if there are sensory findings, foot ulcers, or amputations	At diagnosis, and then annually, or every visit if there are sensory findings, foot ulcers, or amputations
Skin examination, including insulin injection and/or insertion sites	Every visit	Every visit
Psychosocial examination	Annually	Annually

(*Adapted from* the American Diabetes Association. Comprehensive Medical Evaluation and Assessment of Comorbidities: Standards of Medical Care in Diabetes- 2021. Diabetes Care 2021 Jan; 44(Supplement 1): S40-S52).

assessment on examination for depression, anxiety, as well as disordered eating and cognitive capacities using patient-appropriate standardized and validated tools.[35]

A starting point for practitioners may be in asking whether the patient has noted changes in mood since the last clinical visit. Assessment of any new obstacles to treatment and self-management, including stress from diabetes or other life stressors may be an integral part of the examination. Caregivers and family members may benefit from being included in the provider's psychosocial examination.

SUMMARY

This review of the physical examination in patients with diabetes highlights the importance of routine and repeat examination to identify diagnostic and macro-/microvascular complications that can occur during the course of the disease of patients with type 1 and type 2 DM. **Table 2** describes the significant components of physical examination and recommended frequency of examinations. To support the goal of providing comprehensive care to patients with diabetes, in addition to the physical examination, providers should also be routinely assessing medical history, laboratory tests, as well as diabetes self-management behaviors, nutrition, social determinants of health, and psychosocial health.

CLINICS CARE POINTS

- Checking blood pressure at every visit is important to keep blood pressure within the goal of less than 130/80 in patients with diabetes who have a 10-year ASCVD risk of ≥ 15% and less than 140/90 in those with a 10-year ASCVD risk of less than 15%. Orthostatic blood pressure measurements can be checked on initial assessment and subsequently as indicated to detect autonomic dysfunction or hypovolemia caused by osmotic diuresis in patients with diabetes.

- Referral to specialists to detect DR using screening dilated fundus examination or retinal photography is important to identify this condition before it progresses to the proliferative phase and causes macular edema and blindness.
- A foot examination of a patient with diabetes begins with the removal of shoes and socks to perform a visual inspection. From there, detecting peripheral neuropathy using a variety of neurologic tests including the 10 g monofilament test can help prevent diabetic foot ulcers.
- An oral examination to detect periodontitis and gingivitis is often neglected but can assist in improving glycemic control.
- A thorough skin examination can help identify skin changes at the insertion sites of insulin pumps and CGM sensors. Preventing device-related infections and improving patient adherence in the use of diabetes technology supports the effective management of diabetes.

DISCLOSURE

The authors have nothing to disclose.

REFERENCES

1. Dieleman JL, Baral R, Birger M, et al. US spending on personal health care and public health, 1996-2013. JAMA 2016;316(24):2627–46.
2. https://www.cdc.gov/diabetes/data/statistics-report/diagnosed-undiagnosed-diabetes.html. Accessed July 31, 2021.
3. Xie X, Atkins E, Lv J, et al. Effects of intensive blood pressure lowering on cardiovascular and renal outcomes: updated systematic review and meta-analysis. Lancet 2016;387(10017):435.
4. American Diabetes Association. Comprehensive medical evaluation and assessment of comorbidities: standards of medical care in diabetes- 2021. Diabetes Care 2021;44(Supplement 1):S40–52.
5. American Diabetes Association, Position Statement. Treatment of hypertension in adults with diabetes. Diabetes Care 2003;26(suppl 1):s80–2.
6. Whelton PK, Carey RM, Aronow WS, et al. 2017 ACC/AHA/AAPA/ABC/ACPM/AGS/APhA/ASH/ASPC/NMA/PCNA guideline for the prevention, detection, evaluation, and management of high blood pressure in adults: a report of the American college of cardiology/American heart association task force on clinical practice guidelines. Hypertension 2018;71(6):e13.
7. Handelsman Y, Bloomgarden ZT, Grunberger G, et al. American association of clinical endocrinologists and American college of endocrinology—clinical practice guidelines for developing a diabetes mellitus comprehensive care plan—2015. Endocr Pract 2015;21(suppl 1):1–87.
8. American Diabetes Association. Cardiovascular disease and risk management: standards of medical care in diabetes-2021. Diabetes Care 2021; 44(Supplement 1):S125–50.
9. de Boer IH, Bangalore S, Benetos A, et al. Diabetes and hypertension: a position statement by the american diabetes association. Diabetes Care 2017;40(9):1273.
10. Finkelstein EA, Khavjou OA, Thompson H, et al. Obesity and severe obesity forecasts through 2030. Am J Prev Med 2012;42:563–70.

11. Willett WC, Dietz WH, Colditz GA. Guidelines for healthy weight. N Engl J Med 1999;341:427.
12. Knowler WC, Barrett-Connor E, Fowler SE, et al, Diabetes Prevention Program Research Group. Reduction in the incidence of type 2 diabetes with lifestyle intervention or metformin. N Engl J Med 2002;346(6):393.
13. American Diabetes Association. Microvascular complications and foot care: standards of medical care in diabetes-2020. Diabetes Care 2021;44(Suppl 1):S151–67.
14. Taylor CR, Merin LM, Salunga AM, et al. Improving diabetic retinopathy screening ratios using telemedicine-based digital retinal imaging technology: the Vine Hill study. Diabetes Care 2007;30(3):574.
15. Ahmed J, Ward TP, Bursell SE, et al. The sensitivity and specificity of nonmydriatic digital stereoscopic retinal imaging in detecting diabetic retinopathy. Diabetes Care 2006;29(10):2205.
16. O'Hare JP, Hopper A, Madhaven C, et al. Adding retinal photography to screening for diabetic retinopathy: a prospective study in primary care. BMJ 1996;312(7032):679.
17. Teshome A, Yitayeh A. The effect of periodontal therapy on glycemic control and fasting plasma glucose level in type 2 diabetic patients: systematic review and meta-analysis. BMC Oral Health 2016;17(1):31.
18. Hein C. Scottsdale revisited: the role of dental practitioners in screening for undiagnosed diabetes and the medical co-management of patients with diabetes or those at risk for diabetes. Compend Contin Educ Dent 2008;29(9):538.
19. Melmed S, Koenig R, Rosen C, et al. Williams textbook of endocrinology. 14th edition. Philadelphia: Elsevier; 2020. p. 1519.
20. Armstrong DG, Boulton AJM, Bus SA. Diabetic foot ulcers and their recurrence. N Engl J Med 2017;376:2367.
21. Walsh JW, Hoffstad OJ, Sullivan MO, et al. Association of diabetic foot ulcer and death in a population-based cohort from the United Kingdom. Diabet Med 2016; 33:1493.
22. Ndip A, Lavery LA, Lafontaine J, et al. High levels of foot ulceration and amputation risk in a multiracial cohort of diabetic patients on dialysis therapy. Diabetes Care 2010;33(4):878–80.
23. Boulton AJ, Armstrong DG, Albert SF, et al. Comprehensive foot examination and risk assessment: a report of the task force of the foot care interest group of the American Diabetes Association, with endorsement by the American Association of Clinical Endocrinologists. Diabetes Care 2008;31(8):1679–85.
24. Kanji JN, Anglin RES, Hunt DL, et al. Does this patient with diabetes have large-fiber peripheral neuropathy? JAMA 2010;303(15):1526–32.
25. Shahzad M, Al Robaee A, Al Shobaili HA, et al. Skin manifestations in diabetic patients attending a diabetic clinic in the Qassim region, Saudi Arabia. Med Princ Pract 2011;20:137–41.
26. Mahmood T, Bari A, Agha H. Cutaneous manifestations of diabetes mellitus. J Pakistan Assoc Dermatologists 2005;15:227–32.
27. Murphy-Chutorian B, Han G, Cohen SR. Dermatologic manifestations of diabetes mellitus: a review. Endocrinol Metab Clin North Am 2013;42:869.
28. Morgan AJ, Schwartz RA. Diabetic dermopathy: a subtle sign with grave implications. J Am Acad Dermatol 2008;58:447.
29. Dawber RP. Vitiligo in mature-onset diabetes mellitus. Br J Dermatol 1968;80: 275–8.
30. Gould IM, Gray RS, Urbaniak SJ, et al. Vitiligo in diabetes mellitus. Br J Dermatol 1985;113:153–5.

31. Afkhami-Ardekani M, Ghadiri-Anari A, Ebrahimzadeh-Ardakani M, et al. Prevalence of vitiligo among type 2 diabetic patients in an Iranian population. Int J Dermatol 2014;53(8):956–8.
32. Raveendra L, Hemavathi RN, Rajgopal S. A study of vitiligo in type 2 diabetic patients. Indian J Dermatol 2017;62(2):168–70.
33. Cheng J, Kuai D, Zhang L, et al. Psoriasis increased the risk of diabetes: a meta-analysis. Arch Dermatol Res 2012;304:119–25.
34. American Diabetes Association. Facilitating behavior change and well-being to improve health outcomes: standards of medical care in diabetes—2021. Diabetes Care 2021;44(Supplement 1):S53–72.
35. Young-Hyman D, de Groot M, Hill-Briggs F, et al. Psychosocial care for people with diabetes: a position statement of the American diabetes association. Diabetes Care 2016;39:2126–40.

Endocrinopathies

Dana Sheely, MD*, Deepti Pujare, MD

KEYWORDS

- Cushing disease • adrenal insufficiency • hypothyroidism • hyperthyroidism
- thyroid nodules • polycystic ovarian syndrome

KEY POINTS

- Important features of Cushing syndrome include purple abdominal striae, facial plethora, buffalo hump, proximal muscle weakness, central obesity, and diabetes mellitus.
- Primary adrenal insufficiency can present with hypotension, hyperpigmentation, fatigue, and gastrointestinal symptoms such as nausea and vomiting.
- Findings in patients with hypothyroidism can include goiter, weight gain, bradycardia, and delayed deep tendon reflexes.
- Patients with hyperthyroidism present with tremor, hyperreflexia, tachycardia, and orbitopathy.
- Patients with polycystic ovary syndrome present with oligomenorrhea, hyperandrogenism, and features of metabolic syndrome such as weight gain and diabetes mellitus.

CUSHING SYNDROME

Introduction and Definition

Cushing syndrome is caused by prolonged exposure to inappropriately elevated levels of plasma glucocorticoids. It can occur due to endogenous or exogenous sources. Endogenous sources can be either adrenocorticotropic hormone (ACTH) independent or ACTH dependent. ACTH-independent sources include cortisol-producing adrenal adenomas. ACTH-dependent sources include pituitary adenomas or ectopic ACTH-producing tumors. Exogenous sources can include prolonged systemic or topical corticosteroid use.

Discussion

Patients are screened for Cushing syndrome based on certain signs and symptoms. Some of the signs of Cushing syndrome, such as hyperglycemia and truncal obesity, overlap with those found commonly in the general population, and it is therefore important to perform a comprehensive history and physical examination in patients

Division of Endocrinology, Diabetes and Metabolism, University of California, Davis, 4150 V Street, PSSB G400, Sacramento, CA 95817, USA
* Corresponding author.
E-mail address: dmsheely@ucdavis.edu

Med Clin N Am 106 (2022) 495–507
https://doi.org/10.1016/j.mcna.2021.12.010

suspected of having this syndrome. These patients typically have progressively worsening signs and symptoms over time.

Patients with Cushing syndrome can have findings such as central obesity that involves the face, neck, trunk, and abdomen. This appearance is different from generalized obesity, which is more common in the population. Other features of metabolic syndrome, including type 2 diabetes mellitus and hypertension, may also be present. A common finding in Cushing syndrome is rounding of the face due to fat accumulation in the cheeks, which is termed "moon facies." Patients may also develop facial plethora—a fullness of the face with a flushed appearing or reddish complexion. These patients often develop fat deposits over the thoraco-cervical spine (termed "buffalo hump") and in the supraclavicular fossae (**Fig. 2**).

Dermatologic manifestations of Cushing syndrome include a virtually pathognomonic sign of the presence of this syndrome which are purple, nonblanching striae that can be found on the abdomen, arms, and thighs. These striae are usually more than 1 cm in width and look different from the pale striae that occur in pregnant women or in the setting of rapid weight gain or loss (**Fig. 1**).[1] Women with Cushing syndrome can develop signs of hyperandrogenism because the adrenal glands are the main source of androgen production in women. These signs include hirsutism with particularly marked hair growth on the upper lip and chin. Other dermatologic findings include easy bruising as well as thinning of the skin due to prolonged corticosteroid exposure. Another feature of Cushing syndrome includes wrinkling of the skin on the dorsal surface of the hand, which results in a "cigarette paper" appearance known as Liddle sign.[1]

Musculoskeletal manifestations of Cushing syndrome include proximal muscle weakness involving the upper or lower extremities manifested by difficulty rising from a seated position, climbing stairs, or raising the hands above the head. Osteoporosis may occur resulting in bone loss followed by fragility and vertebral compression fractures and resultant loss in height.

The cardiovascular signs of hypercortisolism may include hypertension, and severe hypercortisolism can even cause a hypercoaguable state resulting in physical findings consistent with deep vein thrombosis or pulmonary embolism. **Table 1** lists some of the highest yield findings for Cushing syndrome.[2]

ADRENAL INSUFFICIENCY
Introduction and Definition

Adrenal insufficiency refers to glucocorticoid deficiency with or without concurrent mineralocorticoid deficiency and adrenal androgen deficiency and can be primary, secondary, or tertiary in origin. Primary adrenal insufficiency refers to disease that occurs in the adrenal cortex, whereas secondary adrenal insufficiency occurs due to pituitary disease leading to decreased secretion of ACTH. Tertiary adrenal insufficiency results from impaired release of corticotropin-releasing hormone from the hypothalamus, which then fails to stimulate the secretion of ACTH from the pituitary gland. The causes of primary, secondary, and tertiary adrenal insufficiency are summarized in **Boxes 1–3**.[3]

A key difference between primary adrenal insufficiency and secondary or tertiary adrenal insufficiency is that primary adrenal insufficiency results in mineralocorticoid deficiency, whereas secondary and tertiary adrenal insufficiencies do not. This is because aldosterone secretion is regulated by the renin-angiotensin-aldosterone system (RAAS) and not by the pituitary gland. In secondary and tertiary adrenal insufficiency, only glucocorticoid secretion from the adrenal gland is affected.

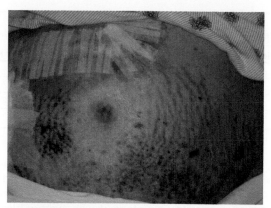

Fig. 1. Abdominal striae and bruising in a patient with Cushing syndrome (with permission from the collection of P. Aronowitz).

Discussion

Adrenal insufficiency can be chronic in nature or can present acutely, as an adrenal crisis, which is a life-threatening emergency. Chronic adrenal insufficiency presents with nonspecific signs and symptoms that can lead to a delay in diagnosis. Symptoms related to glucocorticoid deficiency include fatigue, weight loss, abdominal pain, nausea, and vomiting. Mineralocorticoid deficiency causes dizziness, orthostatic

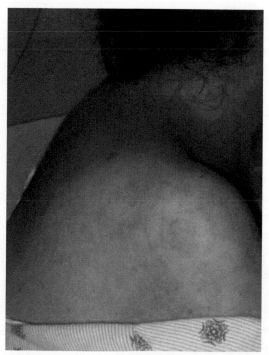

Fig. 2. Dorsocervical hump in a patient with Cushing syndrome (with permission from the collection of P. Aronowitz).

Table 1
Findings with increased likelihood ratios predicting the presence of Cushing syndrome

Physical Examination Finding	Likelihood Ratio if Finding Is Present
Skin thinning	115.6
Bruising	4.5
Central obesity	3.0
Facial plethora	2.7

hypotension, and, sometimes, salt craving. Adrenal androgen deficiency is more pronounced in women and can cause symptoms such as dry skin and loss of libido.

Patients with adrenal insufficiency may present with several key physical examination findings and are often relatively hypotensive with systolic blood pressures less than 100 mm Hg. Orthostatic hypotension due to mineralocorticoid deficiency may also be present. Weight loss due to volume depletion and anorexia are also often present. Patients with primary adrenal insufficiency may have skin hyperpigmentation, which occurs due to increased production of proopiomelanocortin, a prohormone that is cleaved into ACTH, melanocyte-stimulating hormone (MSH), and other hormones. The elevated MSH leads to increased melanin synthesis, which leads to hyperpigmentation. Brown pigmentation can be diffuse but tends to be more obvious in sun-exposed areas of the face, neck, and back of the hands. It also can be prominent in the palmar creases, on the inner surface of the lips, and the buccal mucosa.[1] Skin hyperpigmentation is an important distinguishing characteristic between primary and secondary adrenal insufficiency because it does not occur in patients with secondary adrenal insufficiency.

Primary adrenal insufficiency may occur in the context of autoimmune polyendocrinopathy syndromes. There are two predominant types of autoimmune polyglandular syndromes (APS type 1 and type 2). APS type 1 (abbreviated as APECED) is associated with Addison disease, chronic mucocutaneous candidiasis, ectodermal dystrophy, and hypoparathyroidism. It is caused by mutations in the *AIRE* gene and is

Box 1
Causes of primary adrenal insufficiency

Autoimmune adrenalitis caused by 21-21-hydroxylase autoantibodies hydro

APS type 1 (*AIRE* gene mutation)

APS type 2

Infectious adrenalitis (tuberculosis, HIV, fungal, and other infections)

Genetic disorders (adrenoleukodystrophy)

Adrenal metastases

Adrenal hemorrhage

Adrenal infarction

Medications (fluconazole, ketoconazole, phenytoin, etomidate, and others)

Congenital adrenal hypoplasia

Congenital adrenal hyperplasia

Familial glucocorticoid resistance

Box 2
Causes of secondary adrenal insufficiency

Pituitary tumors

Pituitary trauma

Pituitary surgery

Pituitary radiation therapy

Infections or abscesses (tuberculosis and others)

Infiltrative processes (sarcoidosis, lymphocytic hypophysitis, hemochromatosis, and others)

Pituitary infarction

Pituitary apoplexy

Genetic mutations (eg, *HESX1* gene mutation)

---

inherited in an autosomal recessive fashion. Important physical examination findings in these patients are mucocutaneous candidiasis and less frequently, candidiasis affecting the esophagus and skin.[4] Ectodermal dystrophy refers to pitted nails and enamel hypoplasia.[4] Physical examination findings of hypoparathyroidism include features of hypocalcemia such as the presence of a Chvostek or Trousseau sign. Primary adrenal insufficiency can also occur in the context of APS type II, which is more common. APS type II is defined by a patient having two or more of the following: Addison disease, autoimmune thyroid disease, type 1 diabetes, primary hypogonadism, and other nonendocrine manifestations (such as myasthenia gravis).[4]

In patients with chronic secondary adrenal insufficiency, only glucocorticoid production is affected, and as a result, these patients have symptoms such as fatigue, anorexia, weight loss, nausea, and generalized abdominal pain. Hyperpigmentation is not present because ACTH production is decreased and hypotension usually does not occur because the RAAS system is intact. Manifestations of a pituitary or hypothalamic tumor may include anterior pituitary hormone deficiencies as well as headaches and visual field deficits if the tumor is causing increased intracranial pressure or compressing the optic chiasm.

Acute adrenal crisis is a medical emergency and needs to be treated immediately with high-dose corticosteroids. Patients with acute adrenal insufficiency present with complaints of fatigue, nausea, vomiting, and abdominal pain. Physical examination is often remarkable for the presence of hypotension, altered level of mentation,

---

Box 3
Causes of tertiary adrenal insufficiency

Hypothalamic masses (craniopharyngiomas or metastases from distant primary cancer)

Traumatic brain injury

Hypothalamic surgery

Hypothalamic irradiation

Infections

Infiltrative processes

Glucocorticoid therapy (systemic, topical, or inhaled steroids)

and generalized abdominal tenderness. Patients may also have a fever due to an increased inflammatory response or the presence of an infection. Patients with acute adrenal insufficiency due to bilateral adrenal hemorrhage or infarction often present with hypotension, abdominal and flank tenderness, and decreased hemoglobin.

HYPOTHYROIDISM
Introduction and Definition

Hypothyroidism refers to thyroid hormone deficiency and can be classified as primary or secondary. In iodine-sufficient areas, the most common cause of primary hypothyroidism is autoimmune thyroiditis, more commonly known as Hashimoto disease. The most common causes of primary and secondary hypothyroidism are listed in **Boxes 4–6** and **Tables 2 and 3.**[5]

Discussion

The manifestations of hypothyroidism can affect all the organ systems. Some of the most common signs and symptoms of hypothyroidism include the following:

- *General:* weight gain, cold intolerance, and fatigue
- *Pulmonary:* dyspnea on exertion
- *Neurologic:* impaired memory and mood impairment
- *Gastrointestinal:* constipation
- *Endocrinologic:* menstrual dysfunction and manifestations of metabolic syndrome including hypertension and dyslipidemia
- *Musculoskeletal:* muscle weakness, muscle cramps, and arthralgias
- *Dermatologic:* coarse skin, alopecia, and brittle nails

Generalized physical examination findings of hypothyroidism include weight gain, bradycardia, and diastolic hypertension. In patients with Hashimoto thyroiditis, the thyroid gland may be firm or rubbery, and the thyroid examination may reveal a goiter in cases of severe hypothyroidism.

Dermatologic manifestations of hypothyroidism include pale, cool skin due to vasoconstriction and anemia. Hair loss, brittle nails, dry skin, and decreased sweating may be present in cases of severe hypothyroidism. Periorbital edema may occur, manifested as a puffy appearance around the eyes due to the accumulation of myxedematous tissue. Edema can also occur on the dorsa of the hands and feet as well as in the supraclavicular fossae.[6,7]

Box 4
Causes of primary hypothyroidism

Autoimmune thyroiditis (Hashimoto thyroiditis)

Iatrogenic (thyroidectomy, radiation)

Thyroiditis (painless thyroiditis, postpartum thyroiditis, and viral thyroiditis)

Drug induced (amiodarone, lithium, and checkpoint inhibitor therapy)

Iodine deficiency

Infiltrative diseases (sarcoidosis and hemochromatosis)

Thyroid malignancy

Metastases to the thyroid gland

Box 5
Causes of secondary hypothyroidism

Pituitary masses causing Thyroid stimulating hormone (TSH) deficiency

Hypothalamic disease causing Thyrotropin-releasing Hormone (TRH) deficiency

Resistance to TSH/TRH

The neurologic examination in the presence of hypothyroidism often reveals delayed relaxation of deep tendon reflexes, and in the elderly population, memory defects and lethargy can be present. Psychiatric manifestations, such as depression and other mood disorders, are frequently associated with hypothyroidism.

Patients with hypothyroidism due to thyroiditis may have characteristic findings on physical examination. Viral thyroiditis usually results in thyroid tenderness (and is often preceded by upper respiratory symptoms). Riedel thyroiditis is rare and occurs due to fibrosis of the thyroid gland, which extends into adjacent tissues. Riedel thyroiditis can present with an enlarged thyroid gland or goiter, which is hard, asymmetric, and fixed to adjacent tissues and muscles. These patients can have compressive symptoms such as hoarseness, shortness of breath, and dysphagia due to fibrosis involving surrounding structures such as the recurrent laryngeal nerve, trachea, and esophagus.

Patients with secondary hypothyroidism due to a pituitary tumor may present with other signs and symptoms of a pituitary adenoma. It is important to screen for coexisting anterior pituitary hormone deficiencies. Patients may also have visual field deficits due to compression of the optic chiasm from the enlarging pituitary tumor.

Box 6
Common causes of hyperthyroidism[8]

Thyrotoxicosis associated with normal or elevated radioiodine uptake

Graves' disease

Hashitoxicosis

Toxic adenoma

Toxic multinodular goiter

TSH-producing pituitary adenoma

HCG-mediated hyperthyroidism

Thyrotoxicosis associated with low radioiodine uptake

Subacute (DeQuervain, granulomatous) thyroiditis

Thyroiditis (lymphocytic thyroiditis and postpartum thyroiditis)

Amiodarone-induced thyroiditis

Thyroiditis induced by checkpoint inhibitors

Radiation thyroiditis

Iatrogenic thyrotoxicosis

Intentional ingestion of thyroid hormone

Struma ovarii

Table 2
Findings with increased likelihood ratios for the presence of hypothyroidism[2]

Physical Examination Finding	Likelihood Ratio if Finding Is Present
Hypothyroid speech (low voice, reduced range, low pitch)	5.4
Bradycardia	4.2
Coarse skin	3.4
Delayed ankle reflexes	3.4

HYPERTHYROIDISM
Introduction and Definition

Hyperthyroidism refers to increased thyroid hormone production by the thyroid gland. Signs and symptoms of hyperthyroidism can affect several organ systems and are listed as follows:

- *General:* weight loss
- *Eyes:*
  - Graves' eye disease can lead to proptosis, lid lag, dry eyes, conjunctival erythema, and irritation
- *Cardiovascular:*
  - Tachycardia, widened pulse pressure, systolic hypertension, and atrial fibrillation
- *Endocrine:*
  - Osteoporosis, dyslipidemia (low high-density lipoprotein), and hyperglycemia
- *Respiratory:*
  - Dyspnea
- *Gastrointestinal:*
  - Diarrhea (better described as soft, formed stools occurring several times each day)
- *Neurologic/psychiatric:*
  - Anxiety, agitation, depression, and psychosis
- *Skin:*
  - Warm skin due to increased blood flow; heat intolerance
  - Sweating, onycholysis, and vitiligo

DISCUSSION

Physical examination findings common to various forms of hyperthyroidism include weight loss due to the hypermetabolic effects of thyroid hormone, systolic hypertension, tachycardia, and irregular heart rhythm due to atrial fibrillation. Some patients

Table 3
Findings with clinically useful positive likelihood ratios for the presence of hyperthyroidism[2]

Physical Examination Finding	Likelihood Ratio if Finding Is Present
Eyelid retraction	33.2
Eyelid lag	18.6
Tremor	11.5
Warm, moist skin	6.8
Tachycardia	4.5

can have systolic hypertension. Neurologic examination often reveals a fine resting tremor, hyperreflexia, and proximal muscle weakness. Dermatologic examination shows warm, moist skin, hair loss, and onycholysis. Pretibial myxedema can occur in more serious cases of hyperthyroidism.

A common cause of hyperthyroidism is Graves' disease, which occurs due to thyroid autoantibodies, either thyroid-stimulating immunoglobulin or TSH receptor antibodies. Patients with Graves' disease have diffuse enlargement of the thyroid gland and a systolic bruit due to markedly increased blood flow to the gland, which may be heard when auscultating over the upper or lower poles of the thyroid gland, where the superior and inferior thyroid arteries enter the gland.[8] Sometimes, a thrill can also be palpated.

Graves' disease causes characteristic findings on eye examination, which include periorbital edema and conjunctival erythema, excessive tearing, and lid retraction, sometimes characterized as "thyroid stare." Examination of extraocular movements may reveal dysconjugate gaze and lid lag. In patients with lid lag, the upper lid lags behind the lobe, exposing more sclera when the patient looks downward or, similarly, when they look upward. Patients with Graves' orbitopathy can have proptosis and exophthalmos which can be measured by an exophthalmometer. Disease activity is assessed using a seven-point clinical activity score, with a score of 3 or more classified as being active disease.

Patients with a toxic adenoma have an autonomously functioning thyroid nodule, and on physical examination, patients may have a palpable thyroid nodule if it is greater than 3 cm in size.[9] Patients with toxic multinodular goiter have an overproduction of thyroid hormone due to multiple hyperfunctioning nodules; however, because these patients produce less thyroid hormone than those with Graves' disease, symptoms are usually milder in nature.[8]

Obstructive symptoms are more common in patients with toxic multinodular goiter than those in Graves' disease due to the characteristics of the thyroid gland.[8] Obstructive symptoms occur due to compression of surrounding cervical structures including the trachea, great vessels, and recurrent laryngeal nerve due to retrosternal extension of the thyroid. Compressive symptoms include dyspnea, dysphagia, hoarseness of voice, or vocal cord paralysis. In rare cases, Horner syndrome may occur due to compression of the cervical sympathetic chain. Toxic multinodular goiter is not usually accompanied by ophthalmologic manifestations and may be a sign of coexistent Graves' disease if also present.[8]

Another cause of hyperthyroidism is subacute thyroiditis which can occur in up to 5% of patients with thyroid disease.[10] Patients with subacute thyroiditis have thyroid pain, swelling, or both often following an upper respiratory infection. On palpation, part of the gland may be enlarged and often tender to palpation and the overlying skin may be warm and erythematous. Other features of a viral infection are commonly present, such as fevers, myalgias, and pharyngitis. Up to 50% of patients have symptoms of thyrotoxicosis.[10] Usually the symptoms are self-limited but can last for several months. In about 90% of patients, no residual deficiency in thyroid function remains after recovery.[8]

Struma ovarii occurs when thyroid tissue is present in ovarian teratomas. Thyrotoxicosis can occur in 8% to 10% of patients.[8] Patients generally present with lower abdominal pain or a mass and can occasionally have ascites. Findings on radioiodine scan indicate low uptake in the thyroid gland. Rarely, women who have a struma ovarii can present with a goiter, and these patients often have coexistent Grave disease.[11]

TSH-secreting adenomas are a rare cause of hyperthyroidism. A case series revealed that about 94% of patients with TSH-secreting pituitary adenomas have a goiter.[12] These patients can have features of hyperthyroidism including palpitations, tremors, weight loss, and heat intolerance. They also have symptoms of a pituitary mass including headaches and visual field deficits such as bitemporal hemianopsia. Because TSH-secreting adenomas may cosecrete growth hormone and prolactin, it is important to assess for physical examination changes related to acromegaly and prolactinoma. In a case series with 255 patients with TSH-secreting adenomas, about 33% had menstrual disturbances and 28% had galactorrhea which are suggestive of prolactin excess.[12] Patients should be screened for findings of acromegaly including enlarged jaw, enlarged hands and feet, and coarse facial features, among other findings.

Hyperthyroidism can present differently in elderly patients as compared with younger patients. In one cross-sectional study, elderly patients had a higher prevalence of weight loss and shortness of breath but were less likely to have typical features of hyperthyroidism such as heat tolerance, anxiety, or tremors.[13] Apathetic hyperthyroidism refers to elderly patients who do not display the classic features of hyperthyroidism. These patients seem depressed or withdrawn and can be misdiagnosed as having psychiatric disorders such as depression or even suspected to have underlying malignancy. Patients with apathetic hyperthyroidism often have staring, placid faces, and weakness and muscle wasting are common in this disorder.[8]

THYROID NODULES
Introduction and Definition

Thyroid nodules are common and can be found in up to 65% of the population.[14] Thyroid nodules can be palpated by the patient, discovered on physical examination, or incidentally found on imaging studies such as computed tomography, magnetic resonance imaging, or ultrasound. Most thyroid nodules are benign, and the incidence of cancer ranges around 5%–10%.[14] Risk factors for cancer include previous head or neck irradiation, family history of thyroid cancer or thyroid cancer syndromes (such as multiple endocrine neoplasia type 2, familial adenomatous polyposis, or Cowden syndrome). Most patients with thyroid nodules are euthyroid and less than 5% of nodules cause hyperthyroidism or thyrotoxicosis.[14]

Discussion

Clinically, most patients with thyroid nodules are asymptomatic. Some patients with large thyroid nodules may complain of compressive symptoms such as dysphagia, dyspnea, dysphonia or hoarseness, whereas others may complain of a globus sensation (the feeling that something is stuck in the throat). Patients who have a globus sensation usually have a nodule greater than 3 cm, and the nodule is likely to be located close to the trachea.[14] Thyroid nodules that lead to dysphagia are located in the left lobe and extend posteriorly leading to compression of the esophagus.[14] Nodules that are increasing rapidly in size or have hemorrhage into them can cause pain. Thyroid nodules that are firm, fixed, rapidly growing, or associated with cervical lymphadenopathy must be evaluated promptly to rule out thyroid cancer.

Some patients with thyroid nodules will have a normal physical examination if the nodules are small or located posteriorly within the gland. On examination of the thyroid gland, it is important to note the size, number, and consistency of the nodules; the presence of multiple thyroid nodules can be a sign of multinodular goiter. Benign nodules tend to be smooth, soft, mobile, and generally do not cause obstructive symptoms. Suspicious nodules are generally hard, fixed, and irregular. When a patient presents with thyroid nodules, it is also imperative to examine the cervical lymph

> **Box 7**
> **Rotterdam criteria to diagnose PCOS**
>
> Rotterdam criteria (Two of the following criteria are required to make the diagnosis):
>   Oligo and/or anovulation
>   Clinical and/or biochemical signs of hyperandrogenism
>   Polycystic ovaries (by ultrasound)

node chains for evidence of lymphadenopathy as the presence of large, firm lymph nodes may indicate the presence of thyroid cancer. In addition to physical examination, thyroid nodules can be further evaluated with thyroid ultrasound.

In patients with obstructive symptoms due to a goiter or multinodular goiter, the examiner can ask the patient to perform the Pemberton maneuver. For this maneuver, the patient raises the arms vertically above the head for about 60 seconds. This test is considered positive (Pemberton sign) if the patient's neck veins become more distended or if the patient develops facial plethora, cyanosis, or dyspnea due to impaired venous return from the neck and face due to compression of the great vessels by the goiter.

POLYCYSTIC OVARY SYNDROME
Introduction and Definition

Polycystic ovary syndrome (PCOS) is an endocrinopathy affecting women and is characterized by a constellation of signs and symptoms. It is characterized by oligomenorrhea, hyperandrogenism, and symptoms of metabolic syndrome. The Rotterdam criteria are used to make a diagnosis of PCOS (**Box 7**).

Discussion

Women with PCOS frequently have oligomenorrhea or amenorrhea, so it is important to take a detailed menstrual cycle history. They often have features of hyperandrogenism such as hirsutism which is characterized by thick terminal hair in a male distribution pattern (upper lip, chin, and periareolar area). Hair growth can be characterized using the Ferriman–Gallwey score to evaluate hirsutism. Women with PCOS also have androgenic alopecia or hair loss pattern seen in men. In rare cases, patients can develop acne, clitoromegaly, deepening of the voice, and oily skin. If women present with these symptoms, other serious causes of hyperandrogenism (such as adrenal or ovarian tumors) should be excluded.

Women who have PCOS can develop insulin resistance leading to hyperglycemia or diabetes mellitus. The insulin resistance can lead to obesity and associated

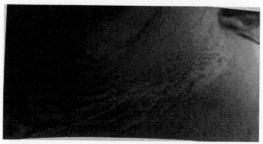

Fig. 3. Acanthosis nigricans on the neck of a patient with PCOS.[18] (With permission from the collection of S. Karakas).

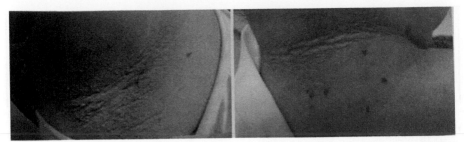

Fig. 4. Skin tags on a patient with PCOS. (With permission from the collection of S. Karakas).

comorbidities of hypertension and dyslipidemia. It is important to check patient's weight, body mass index (BMI), and blood pressure at every visit. A recent study found that women with PCOS are more likely to develop hypertension beginning in early adulthood (by age 35), independent of BMI.[15,16] The study concluded that PCOS was independently associated with 37% greater risk of hypertension when compared with women without PCOS.[15]

Body fat distribution can be assessed by checking waist and hip circumference. Women with PCOS often have a BMI of 30 or higher. Due to increased insulin resistance, patients develop dark skin patches in the axillae, neck, and thighs known as acanthosis nigricans as well as skin tags in these same regions (**Figs. 3** and **4**). Insulin resistance can also lead to nonalcoholic fatty liver disease; it is therefore important to assess for liver size which may be suggestive of hepatomegaly from evolving liver disease.

It is important to screen for obstructive sleep apnea (OSA) in patients with PCOS. One meta-analysis concluded that patients with PCOS are about 9.7 times more likely to develop OSA.[17] Although the exact mechanism of how PCOS leads to OSA has not been elucidated, one important link seems to be the presence of obesity. Obesity can lead to increased fat deposition around the pharynx and decreased thoracic compliance. Patients should be asked about symptoms of sleep apnea such as excessive daytime sleepiness or snoring during sleep.

Finally, women with PCOS can develop psychiatric or mood disorders such as anxiety or depression. Screening for these disorders using a Patient Health Questionaire 9 (PHQ-9) questionnaire should be part of the evaluation for women with PCOS.

CLINICS CARE POINTS

- Cushing syndrome should be considered when there is the presence of violaceous striae.
- Adrenal crisis is a medical emergency that can present similar to septic shock and should be treated with high dose corticosteroids.
- Thyroid nodules are present in up to 65% of the population, however, 90-95% of these nodules are benign.
- Polycystic ovarian syndrome should be considered in women with oligomenorrhea, clinical signs of hyperandrogenism and insulin resistance.

DISCLOSURE

The authors have nothing to disclose.

REFERENCES

1. Melmed S, Auchus RJ, Goldfine AB, et al. In: Williams Textbook of Endocrinology. Philadelphia, (PA): Elsevier; 2020. p. 480–542.
2. McGee S. Evidence-based physical diagnosis e-Book. Elsevier Health Sciences; Web; 2012.
3. Charmandari E, Nicolaides NC, Chrousos GP. Adrenal insufficiency. Lancet 2014; 383(9935):2152–67.
4. Melmed S, Auchus RJ, Goldfine AB, et al. In: Williams Textbook of Endocrinology. Philadelphia, (PA): Elsevier; 2020. p. 1658–71.
5. Chaker L, Bianco AC, Jonklaas J, et al. Hypothyroidism. The Lancet 2017; 390(10101):1550–62.
6. Melmed S, Auchus RJ, Goldfine AB, et al. In: Williams Textbook of Endocrinology. Philadelphia, (PA): Elsevier; 2020. p. 404–32.
7. Ross DS, Burch HB, Cooper DS, et al. 2016 American Thyroid Association Guidelines for Diagnosis and Management of Hyperthyroidism and Other Causes of Thyrotoxicosis. Thyroid 2016;26(10):1343–421.
8. Melmed S, Auchus RJ, Goldfine AB, et al. In: Williams Textbook of Endocrinology. Philadelphia, (PA): Elsevier; 2020. p. 364–403.
9. Siegel RD, Lee SL. Toxic Nodular Goiter. Endocrinol Metab Clin North Am 1998; 27(1):151–68.
10. Pearce EN, Farwell AP, Braverman LE. Thyroiditis. N Engl J Med 2003;348(26): 2646–55.
11. Teale E, Gouldesbrough DR, Peacey SR. Grave Disease and Coexisting Struma Ovarii: Struma Expression of Thyrotropin Receptors and the Presence of Thyrotropin Receptor Stimulating Antibodies. Thyroid 2006;16(8):791–3.
12. Beck-Peccoz P. Thyrotropin-secreting pituitary tumors. Endocr Rev 1996;17(6): 610–38.
13. Trivalle C, Doucet J, Chassagne P, et al. Differences in the Signs and Symptoms of Hyperthyroidism in Older and Younger Patients. J Am Geriatr Soc 1996; 44(1):50–3.
14. Durante C, Grani G, Lamartina L, et al. The Diagnosis and Management of Thyroid Nodules. JAMA 2018;319(9):914.
15. Joham AE, Kakoly NS, Teede HJ, et al. Incidence and Predictors of Hypertension in a Cohort of Australian Women With and Without Polycystic Ovary Syndrome. J Clin Endocrinol Metab 2021;106(6):1585–93.
16. Patel S. Polycystic ovary syndrome (PCOS), an inflammatory, systemic, lifestyle endocrinopathy. J Steroid Biochem Mol Biol 2018;182:27–36.
17. Helvaci N, Karabulut E, Demir AU, et al. Polycystic ovary syndrome and the risk of obstructive sleep apnea: a meta-analysis and review of the literature. Endocr Connections 2017;6(7):437–45.
18. Karakas SE. PCOS: getting the right medical care. United States: The author; 2018.

The Physical Examination to Assess for Anemia and Hypovolemia

Jason D. Napolitano, MD

KEYWORDS

• Anemia • Hemorrhage • Hypovolemia • Volume loss • Physical examination

KEY POINTS

- Supine hypotension, severe orthostatic dizziness, or orthostatic vital sign changes are key indicators of hypovolemia.
- A decreased jugular venous pressure is an insensitive assessment for low central venous pressure.
- Point-of-care ultrasound increases the utility of the bedside examination to assess for hypovolemia.
- Static physical examination maneuvers do not predict volume responsiveness in patients undergoing volume resuscitation, but dynamic maneuvers such as passive leg raising can be useful.
- Specific physical examination findings to search for with anemia include jaundice, splenomegaly, purpura, koilonychia, glossitis, and neurologic findings.

INTRODUCTION

Anemia and hypovolemia are 2 of the most common and most important conditions encountered in clinical medicine. Hypovolemia is defined as a decreased volume of circulating blood in the body.[1] Because the circulating blood volume is made up of approximately 55% plasma and 45% red blood cells, hypovolemia can be caused by acute loss of blood or extracellular fluid volume.[2] Common causes of extracellular fluid volume loss include renal loss from diuresis, gastrointestinal loss from vomiting or diarrhea, insensible water loss through heavy sweating or rapid breathing, and loss of fluid into a "third space," such as the bowel lumen with a bowel obstruction or the peritoneal cavity with ascites. Early diagnosis of hypovolemia is key, as it can lead to initiation of treatment before diminished perfusion leads to end organ damage.

Anemia is a condition in which the number of red blood cells in the body is decreased, although it is tracked by most clinicians with the hemoglobin or hematocrit

David Geffen School of Medicine at UCLA, 757 Westwood Plaza Suite 7501, Los Angeles, CA 90095, USA
E-mail address: jnapolitano@mednet.ucla.edu

Med Clin N Am 106 (2022) 509–518
https://doi.org/10.1016/j.mcna.2021.12.004
0025-7125/22/© 2022 Elsevier Inc. All rights reserved.

on a complete blood count. Anemia can be acute in the setting of hemorrhage. It is important to note that with acute hemorrhage blood and plasma are lost in equal parts. Because of this, the hemoglobin and hematocrit initially remain normal with bleeding, making it important to recognize acute anemia by directly visualizing bleeding or noting findings consistent with bleeding (free fluid in the abdomen, bruising, swollen extremity) and noting physical examination findings consistent with hypovolemia. In this article, we review the uses and limitations of specific physical examination findings to look for hypovolemia.

With chronic anemia, the body has a chance to increase plasma volume to compensate for the loss of red blood cell mass. Physical examination findings suggestive of hypovolemia are often not present, but several classic dermatologic, mucosal, and neurologic findings may suggest both the cause and severity of the anemia. We review key physical examination findings specific to anemia in the second half of the article.

CURRENT EVIDENCE

Many low to medium-quality studies have been done to look at how specific physical examination findings correlate with hypovolemia. Many of the classic findings clinicians are taught in the early stages of their training to look for volume loss have very poor predictive values. For instance, poor skin turgor (slow return of skin to its normal position after being gently pinched by the examiner) does not accurately diagnose hypovolemia in adults.[3,4] In particular, the loss of skin elasticity with aging makes skin turgor particularly difficult to assess in elderly individuals. A prolonged capillary refill time (greater than 2 seconds) only has an 11% sensitivity for detecting a 450-mL blood loss in adults.[5,6]

Other, less commonly taught physical examination maneuvers can provide meaningful diagnostic information. For instance, finding a dry axilla on examination increases the probability of hypovolemia.[7] Like most physical examination findings, the lack of axillary sweat should not be looked at in isolation, as it has only a 50% sensitivity for hypovolemia.[6]

The most studied and used maneuvers to look for hypovolemia are supine and orthostatic vital sign measurements and jugular vein assessment. The utility of these tests is discussed in depth as follows.

EVALUATION
Vital Signs

Arterial blood pressure evaluation is critical when hypovolemia is suspected. If a patient has developed supine hypotension, it is likely that they have lost at least 20% to 25% of their arterial blood volume.[8] As cardiovascular collapse may occur with a 40% loss of blood volume, it is critical to recognize the acuity of a patient who has developed supine hypotension in the setting of hemorrhage.

Orthostatic vital signs are a series of blood pressure and pulse measurements taken when a patient has been supine for 2 minutes followed by repeat measurements after the patient has been standing for 1 minute.[6] When an adult stands, approximately 500 mL of blood volume shifts to the lower extremities. This shift has the potential to unmask previously unrecognized hypovolemia. Orthostatic vital signs are classically considered "positive" when any component of the "30/20/10" rule is satisfied. This refers to an increase in the heart rate of 30 or more, a decrease in systolic blood pressure of 20 or more, or a decrease in diastolic blood pressure of 10 or more with standing for 1 minute when compared with values obtained in the supine position. It is no longer considered necessary to check pulse and blood pressure in the seated position and therefore it needs to be checked only in the supine and standing positions. It is important to note that orthostatic hypotension may be present at baseline in nearly 20% of individuals older than 65, decreasing the specificity of this finding.[9] Whereas mild dizziness with standing is not helpful to diagnose hypovolemia, severe dizziness with standing is suggestive of large-volume blood loss.[6]

JUGULAR VENOUS PRESSURE ASSESSMENT

A jugular venous pressure (JVP) below 5 cm of water is suggestive of hypovolemia. To accurately measure the JVP, a patient's bed should be adjusted to an appropriate angle to clearly display the "meniscus" or highest vertical level of pulsation of the internal jugular vein (please see the video demonstrating how to locate the internal jugular vein in **Fig. 1** of the article, "Congestive Heart Failure," elsewhere in this issue). Adjusting the bed to a 30-degree to 45-degree angle is often quoted by teachers of the physical examination. There is nothing magical about this angle. It really just acts as a good starting point for positioning where in most patients the jugular venous pulsations will be above the clavicle and below the angle of the mandible and thus will be able to be visually assessed. At an angle of 45°, the clavicle sits roughly 2 cm vertical to the sternal angle and a patient's JVP will need to be at least 7 cm of water for jugular venous pulsations to be visible above the clavicle. In patients with significant hypovolemia, the angle of the hospital bed or examination table may need to be adjusted to an angle of less than 30° to see internal jugular venous pulsations. Regardless of the positioning of the patient, it is the vertical height of the internal jugular venous pulsations that estimates central venous pressure. This vertical height is measured from the sternal angle, and 5 cm are added to the measured height to account for the average distance from the sternal angle to the center of the right atrium. The measurement of JVP is analogous to the measurement of tire pressure with a tire gauge. Where the pressure within a tire causes the manometer rise against gravity, the pressure in the right atrium causes the blood within the jugular vein to rise vertically against gravity.

Small studies have shown a variable performance of assessment of the JVP to estimate central venous pressure. In one study in which clinicians used visual inspection of the JVP to estimate central venous pressure (CVP), a clinical assessment of low CVP had a positive likelihood (LR+) of 3 that a CVP measured with a central venous

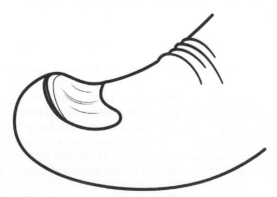

Fig. 1. Illustration of koilonychia demonstrating a concavity in the nail bed giving the appearance of a "spoon-shaped" nail that could hold a drop of water. This finding is often most notable in the first 3 digits.

catheter would be low.[10,11] No patient assessed clinically as having a high CVP ended up having a low CVP on invasive monitoring.[10,11] This could be taken as a bedside rule of thumb that a patient with an elevated JVP is in the vast majority of instances *not hypovolemic*. Notable exceptions could include patients with cor pulmonale or acute right heart failure in the setting of an acute myocardial infarction that involves the right ventricle. In these instances, the JVP may be elevated even in the setting of intravascular hypovolemia. In another separate small study, the sensitivity of the physical examination plus chest radiograph interpretation to predict a low CVP on subsequent right heart catheterization was 33% and the specificity was 73%.[10,12]

It is worth noting that the JVP is more commonly underestimated than overestimated. Although numerous physical examination textbooks state that a "normal" JVP is 5 to 9 cm of water, a normal CVP can vary from person to person and is dependent on numerous factors separate from volume status, including venous tone, intrathoracic pressure, and ventricular compliance. Therefore, even a direct measurement of CVP may not accurately predict volume status. Consequently, when using a JVP estimate at the bedside, a clinician should take into account that a "low" JVP can be seen with hypovolemia but is not by itself diagnostic of hypovolemia. To correlate JVP (measured in centimeters of water or cmH_2O) with central line–measured CVP (measured in millimeters of mercury or mm Hg), the JVP can be multiplied by 0.74.

ALTERNATIVE PHYSICAL EXAMINATION MANEUVERS TO ASSESS CENTRAL VENOUS PRESSURE

Although assessment of the internal jugular vein pulsations is recommended for measurement of JVP, one study suggests that assessment of the height of the external jugular vein can predict CVP, as verified by central venous catheter measurements.[13] In this study, the finding of a low external JVP on examination had a 68% sensitivity and a 94% specificity for hypovolemia.[13]

Assessment for hand vein collapse has also been used to assess volume status. To assess for hand vein collapse, the patient should be supine on an examination table or hospital bed. One arm is then placed below the level of the body to cause engorgement of the hand veins with blood. The examiner slowly lifts the patient's hand, observing and palpating the hand veins to see at which level they collapse. This level is measured against the estimated location of the right atrium (the point at which the fourth intercostal space meets the anterior axillary line).[14] The height at which hand vein collapse is observed has been shown to have a sensitivity of 92% and a negative predictive value of 98% for a low CVP.[14]

ADDING POINT-OF-CARE ULTRASOUND TO THE PHYSICAL EXAMINATION

Use of point-of-care ultrasound (POCUS) is of significant value in augmenting the physical examination for assessment of volume status. For example, in patients undergoing hemodialysis, the use of "dry weights" often misjudged intravascular volume status, leading to bouts of hypotension during hemodialysis sessions for those who were above their "dry weight" but intravascularly euvolemic or hypovolemic.[15] The use of hand-carried ultrasounds to assess inferior vena cava (IVC) diameter and collapsibility before deciding how much volume to remove with hemodialysis significantly decreased episodes of hypotension, chest pain, and cramping during dialysis sessions.[15]

To assess volume status using POCUS of the IVC, the IVC diameter should be measured 2 cm from the junction of the IVC and right atrium. An IVC diameter of less than 2 cm correlates with a CVP of less than 10 mm Hg with a sensitivity of

85% and a specificity of 87%.[16] The decrease in IVC diameter during inspiration (in a patient breathing spontaneously) also can be used to gauge volume status. A decrease in IVC diameter of at least 50% during a respiratory cycle can predict a CVP of less than 8 mm Hg with a sensitivity of 91% and a specificity of 94%.[17] Of note, POCUS measurements of the IVC can be rendered inaccurate in the setting of valvular regurgitation, pulmonary hypertension, and right heart failure.

POCUS also can be used to better visualize the apex of the internal jugular venous pulsation. To do this, the patient should be positioned at a 45-degree angle and asked to suspend respiration at the end of exhalation. The ultrasound should then be used to find the height of the a-wave in the internal jugular vein (the level at which the vein tapers).[18] From there, the standard method to measure JVP is used (add 5 cm to the vertical height at which the JVP is measured above the sternal angle). This technique for ultrasound-assisted JVP measurement has a sensitivity of 89% and a specificity of 77% with a negative predictive value of 96% when looking for hypovolemia.[18]

SERIAL ASSESSMENTS OF VOLUME STATUS DURING FLUID RESUSCITATION

Much of the data on using physical examination to detect hypovolemia center on an initial assessment of volume status. In many instances (for example, septic shock with a component of volume depletion), the clinician is called on to make serial assessments of volume status to determine whether additional fluid resuscitation is indicated. Making the correct call in this instance can lead to clinical stabilization of the patient. Approximately 50% of hemodynamically unstable patients with hypotension or signs of organ malperfusion will improve with fluid administration.[19] Administering additional intravenous fluids for a patient in shock who is no longer hypovolemic can lead to fluid overload, with the most important consequence being pulmonary edema. Traditional physical examination findings are of unproven use when assessing a hemodynamically unstable patient for fluid responsiveness.[19]

Studies looking at the performance characteristics of physical examination findings to predict fluid responsiveness in hemodynamically unstable patients are small and have been performed with unique populations of patients. In an observational study of 28 adults with severe malaria, a low JVP, dry mucous membranes, dry axillae, altered tissue turgor, prolonged capillary refill, and tachycardia all had a positive predictive value for volume responsiveness of ≤50%.[20] In the same study, a decreased mean arterial pressure was insensitive at detecting patients with hypovolemia as determined by invasive hemodynamic monitoring. Another study of 28 patients in an intensive care unit asked 2 clinicians to estimate whether they thought patients would be volume responsive based on inspection of the tongue, looking for collapse of the veins on the back of the hand with arm elevation above heart level, examining capillary refill time, inspection of the external jugular vein, and lung auscultation.[21] In 13 of 31 patients, the examiners disagreed on whether the individual would be fluid responsive. In fact, agreement on most of the findings was close to random. The global assessment of whether a patient would be volume responsive based on physical examination in this study was only 37.5% accurate.[21] It should be noted that patients were enrolled in this study after admission to the intensive care unit, and those with obvious hemorrhagic shock were excluded. It is possible that the initial assessment for hypovolemia by physical examination may be of more utility than repeat assessments after initial volume resuscitation has been administered.

Adding the use of POCUS to the physical examination of a patient who needs serial assessments to predict responsiveness to ongoing volume resuscitation may provide additional useful information. In a small study that looked at the collapse of the IVC in spontaneously breathing patients with inspiration, those patients who had a collapse of 40% or more were more likely to respond to additional fluid resuscitation, but not meeting the 40% collapse criteria did not rule out volume responsiveness.[22] The best way to use these findings might be to incorporate IVC measurement into multiple parameters assessed in a given patient. In those with inspiratory collapse of greater than 40%, further volume resuscitation is likely needed. In those without a marked inspiratory IVC collapse, fluid resuscitation still may be indicated depending on the assessment of other clinical data.

A passive leg raise can aid in assessing volume responsiveness. To do this maneuver, the patient is repositioned from semi-recumbent to supine position with the legs elevated to 45°. This leads to movement of approximately 300 mL of venous blood into the central circulation.[23] Some refer to this maneuver as a "self fluid challenge." Although the response to the passive leg raise is best assessed with echocardiographic or esophageal Doppler measurement of changes in cardiac output within 60 seconds of leg raising, an increase of pulse pressure of at least 10% can suggest volume responsiveness with a positive likelihood ratio of 3.6.[19]

PHYSICAL EXAMINATION FINDINGS SPECIFIC FOR ANEMIA

Although the preceding discussion pertains to hypovolemia due to both extracellular fluid loss and hemorrhage, it is worthwhile to consider physical examination findings to assess both acute and chronic anemia. Because acute anemia can be due to a worsening of an underlying pathology that has caused chronic anemia, a careful physical examination will sometimes provide clues as to underlying cause and pace of a patient's disease.

The symptoms a patient may experience due to anemia generally depends on the rate at which the anemia has developed. With acute hemorrhage, symptoms are related to the degree of hypovolemia experienced. If anemia develops gradually, it is usually very well tolerated in patients without underlying cardiac or pulmonary pathology. Even severe anemia with a hemoglobin as low as 5 g/dL can cause minimal symptoms if extracellular fluid volume is maintained (isovolemic anemia).[24] The experiment that proved this concept was done in an operating room where blood was removed by phlebotomy to get volunteers' hemoglobin levels down to approximately 5 g/dL and volume was replaced with plasma and albumin infusions. In the setting of a slow, chronic bleed, the body can compensate in a similar way by retaining extracellular volume and turning it into intravascular volume. When asking patients about symptoms that could be related to anemia, it is worth noting that in the preceding study, the only symptom otherwise healthy patients with marked isovolemic anemia noted while at rest was fatigue.

Patients with iron deficiency anemia may note cravings for clay, dirt, and rocks, which is consistent with pica. They may have an intense desire to eat ice, which is known as pagophagia. A history of visible blood in vomitus, stool, or urine can suggest iron deficiency anemia, as can a history of black stools, which is usually a sign of bleeding proximal to the ligament of Treitz.

There are several physical examination findings the clinician can look for in either the setting of suspected anemia or in the setting of confirmed anemia of unknown etiology. Most have learned to "look directly at capillary beds" by viewing everted lower eyelids, nail beds, or the palmar creases for pallor in the setting of suspected anemia. Pallor is not sensitive for anemia, even when it is severe. In one study, clinical assessment for pallor identified only 61% of severely anemic individuals with a hemoglobin of less than 7 g/dL.[25] However, when pallor is present, it carries clinical significance.

Conjunctival rim pallor has a positive likelihood ratio for anemia of 16.7 and palmar pallor has a positive likelihood ratio for anemia of 5.6.[26]

Clues as to a specific cause of anemia may include concave nail dystrophy, or spoon-shaped nails (koilonychia) with iron deficiency anemia (**Fig. 1**). Koilonychia is present in roughly half of patients with Plummer-Vinson syndrome, which is a triad of iron deficiency anemia, dysphagia, and esophageal webs, which is important to identify given its association with aerodigestive squamous cell carcinomas.[27] Of note, koilonychia does not always represent iron deficiency anemia. It also can be seen with psoriasis, onychomycosis, and trauma.[27] Koilonychia is also insensitive for anemia, occurring in 5.4% of patients with iron deficiency versus 49% of patients with hemochromatosis and up to 29% of cases of hyperthyroidism in one series.[27] The most common nail change with iron depletion is nail brittleness.[28]

Other findings to look for in a patient with anemia include conjunctival icterus with hemolytic anemias, glossitis with iron deficiency or vitamin B12 deficiency anemia, frontal bossing with thalassemia, or splenic enlargement with both hemolytic anemias and conditions such as portal hypertension that are associated with hypersplenism (**Table 1**). Petechiae and purpura can be seen with autoimmune hemolytic anemia and thrombocytopenia (Evans syndrome) and hemolytic uremic syndrome. Multiple myeloma complicated by amyloidosis can cause anemia and is associated with "amyloid purpura" above the nipples, possibly related to amyloid infiltration into blood vessel walls and binding of amyloid proteins to factor X.[29] In particular, amyloid light-chain amyloidosis is associated with periorbital ecchymoses (raccoon eyes) or eyelid purpura.

If anemia is due to vitamin B12 deficiency, many of the examination clues to this diagnosis will be found on the neurologic examination because of the association of

Table 1
Association of specific physical examination findings with etiology of anemia

Etiology of Anemia	Physical Examination Findings
Iron deficiency	Pallor (conjunctival, nail bed, palmar creases) Glossitis Koilonychia Brittle nails
Hemolytic	Conjunctival icterus Enlarged spleen Petechiae and purpura (Evans syndrome and hemolytic uremic syndrome)
Vitamin B12 deficiency	Cognitive dysfunction Weakness Impaired position sense Ataxia Romberg test positive Lhermitte sign
Thalassemia	Hepatosplenomegaly Conjunctival icterus Frontal bossing Shortened arms
Multiple myeloma with amyloid light-chain amyloidosis	Amyloid purpura Periorbital ecchymoses (raccoon eyes)
Hypersplenism	Enlarged spleen Findings of portal hypertension (abdominal wall collateral vessels)

the deficiency with subacute combined degeneration of the spinal cord, which demyelinates the dorsal and lateral columns of the spinal cord. Key physical examination findings with vitamin B12 deficiency include cognitive dysfunction, weakness, abnormal sensation, impaired position sense, ataxia, and a positive Romberg test. Lhermitte sign is the feeling of an "electrical sensation" spreading down the back to the limbs when the patient bends the head forward. This sign can be associated with B12 deficiency and involvement of the posterior columns.

CLINICS CARE POINTS

- Supine hypotension in the setting of hypovolemia represents a loss of at least 20% of the arterial blood volume and requires immediate and aggressive treatment.
- Orthostatic vital signs revealing a rise in pulse of at least 30 beats per minute, a drop in systolic blood pressure of 20 mm Hg or diastolic blood pressure of 10 mm Hg, or severe dizziness with standing have utility in detecting hypovolemia.
- Finding a low JVP is more specific than it is sensitive for hypovolemia, although both sensitivity and specificity are relatively poor.
- A patient with an elevated JVP is usually not hypovolemic.
- Assessment of the external jugular vein and the hand veins are supplemental examination maneuvers used to look for hypovolemia.
- POCUS can improve the accuracy of the physical examination for estimating CVP, with inspiratory collapse of the IVC of at least 50% being the most accurate ultrasound test to look for hypovolemia.
- Static physical examination findings do not help predict which hypovolemic patients who have already received a degree of volume resuscitation will respond to additional fluid administration.
- Increase in pulse pressure with passive leg raise or "self fluid challenge" can suggest continued fluid responsiveness in patients who are being volume resuscitated.
- Vital signs are often normal in patients with chronic anemia.
- Careful dermatologic, mucous membrane, and neurologic examinations can help identify the etiology and important sequelae of chronic anemia.

DISCLOSURE

The author has nothing to disclose.

REFERENCES

1. Merriam-Webster dictionary. Available at: https://www.merriam-webster.com/dictionary/hypovolemia. August 22, 2021.
2. Vaden SL. Blood components. In: American Red Cross blood services. Available at: https://www.redcrossblood.org/donate-blood/how-to-donate/types-of-blood-donations/blood-components.html. August 22, 2021.
3. Gross CR, Lindquist RD, Woolley AC, et al. Clinical indicators of dehydration severity in elderly patients. J Emerg Med 1992;10:267–74.
4. Levitt MA, Lopez B, Lieberman ME, et al. Evaluation of the tilt test in an adult emergency medicine population. Ann Emerg Med 1992;21:713–8.
5. Schriger DL, Baraff LJ. Capillary refill: is it a useful predictor of hypovolemic states? Ann Emerg Med 1991;20:601–5.

6. McGee S, Abernethy WB 3rd, Simel DL. The rational clinical examination. Is this patient hypovolemic? JAMA 1999;281(11):1022–9. https://doi.org/10.1001/jama.281.11.1022.

7. Eaton D, Bannister P, Mulley GP, et al. Axillary sweating in clinical assessment of dehydration in ill elderly patients. BMJ 1994;308:1271.

8. Levy MM, Fink MP, Marshall JC, et al. SCCM/ESICM/ACCP/ATS/SIS. 2001 SCCM/ESICM/ACCP/ATS/SIS international sepsis definitions conference. Crit Care Med 2003;31(4):1250–6. https://doi.org/10.1097/01.CCM.0000050454.01978.3B.

9. Rutan GH, Hermanson B, Bild DE, et al. Orthostatic hypotension in older adults. The Cardiovascular Health Study. CHS Collaborative Research Group. Hypertension 1992;19(6 Pt 1):508–19. https://doi.org/10.1161/01.hyp.19.6.508.

10. Cook DJ, Simel DL. The Rational Clinical Examination. Does this patient have abnormal central venous pressure? JAMA 1996;275(8):630–4.

11. Cook DJ. Clinical assessment of central venous pressure in the critically ill. Am J Med Sci 1990;299(3):175–8. https://doi.org/10.1097/00000441-199003000-00006.

12. Connors AF Jr, McCaffree DR, Gray BA. Evaluation of right-heart catheterization in the critically ill patient without acute myocardial infarction. N Engl J Med 1983;308(5):263–7. https://doi.org/10.1056/NEJM198302033080508.

13. Vinayak AG, Levitt J, Gehlbach B, et al. Usefulness of the external jugular vein examination in detecting abnormal central venous pressure in critically ill patients. Arch Intern Med 2006;166(19):2132–7. https://doi.org/10.1001/archinte.166.19.2132.

14. Vogel F, Staub D, Aschwanden M, et al. Bedside hand vein inspection for noninvasive central venous pressure assessment. Am J Emerg Med 2020;38(2):247–51. https://doi.org/10.1016/j.ajem.2019.04.044.

15. Brennan JM, Ronan A, Goonewardena S, et al. Handcarried ultrasound measurement of the inferior vena cava for assessment of intravascular volume status in the outpatient hemodialysis clinic. Clin J Am Soc Nephrol 2006;1(4):749–53. https://doi.org/10.2215/CJN.00310106.

16. Prekker ME, Scott NL, Hart D, et al. Point-of-care ultrasound to estimate central venous pressure: a comparison of three techniques. Crit Care Med 2013;41(3):833–41. https://doi.org/10.1097/CCM.0b013e31827466b7.

17. Nagdev AD, Merchant RC, Tirado-Gonzalez A, et al. Emergency department bedside ultrasonographic measurement of the caval index for noninvasive determination of low central venous pressure. Ann Emerg Med 2010;55(3):290–5.

18. Siva B, Hunt A, Boudville N. The sensitivity and specificity of ultrasound estimation of central venous pressure using the internal jugular vein. J Crit Care 2012;27(3). https://doi.org/10.1016/j.jcrc.2011.09.008.

19. Bentzer P, Griesdale DE, Boyd J, et al. Will this hemodynamically unstable patient respond to a bolus of intravenous fluids? JAMA 2016;316(12):1298–309. https://doi.org/10.1001/jama.2016.12310.

20. Hanson J, Lam SW, Alam S, et al. The reliability of the physical examination to guide fluid therapy in adults with severe falciparum malaria: an observational study. Malar J 2013;12:348. https://doi.org/10.1186/1475-2875-12-348.

21. Saugel B, Kirsche SV, Hapfelmeier A, et al. Prediction of fluid responsiveness in patients admitted to the medical intensive care unit. J Crit Care 2013;28(4):537.e1–9. https://doi.org/10.1016/j.jcrc.2012.10.008.

22. Muller L, Bobbia X, Toumi M, et al. Respiratory variations of inferior vena cava diameter to predict fluid responsiveness in spontaneously breathing patients

with acute circulatory failure: need for a cautious use. Crit Care 2012;16(5):R188. https://doi.org/10.1186/cc11672.

23. Monnet X, Teboul JL. Passive leg raising: five rules, not a drop of fluid. Crit Care 2015;19(1):18. https://doi.org/10.1186/s13054-014-0708-5.

24. Weiskopf RB, Viele MK, Feiner J, et al. Human cardiovascular and metabolic response to acute, severe isovolemic anemia [published correction appears in JAMA 1998 Oct 28;280(16):1404]. JAMA 1998;279(3):217–21. https://doi.org/10.1001/jama.279.3.217.

25. Montresor A, Albonico M, Khalfan N, et al. Field trial of a haemoglobin colour scale: an effective tool to detect anaemia in preschool children. Trop Med Int Health 2000;5(2):129–33. https://doi.org/10.1046/j.1365-3156.2000.00520.x.

26. Lee AQ, Aronowitz P. Conjunctival and palmar pallor [published online ahead of print, 2021 Jun 25]. J Gen Intern Med 2021. https://doi.org/10.1007/s11606-021-06981-5.

27. Walker J, Baran R, Vélez N, et al. Koilonychia: an update on pathophysiology, differential diagnosis and clinical relevance. J Eur Acad Dermatol Venereol 2016; 30(11):1985–91. https://doi.org/10.1111/jdv.13610.

28. Sobolewski S, Lawrence AC, Bagshaw P. Human nails and body iron. J Clin Pathol 1978;31(11):1068–72. https://doi.org/10.1136/jcp.31.11.1068.

29. Kelsey A, Smith DH, Meng J, et al. Amyloidosis: a story of how inframammary erosions eclipsed inconspicuous periorbital ecchymoses. Int J Womens Dermatol 2016;2(1):18–22. https://doi.org/10.1016/j.ijwd.2015.11.001.

Movement Disorders

Daniel Winkel, MD[a],*, Lisa Bernstein, MD, FACP[b]

KEYWORDS

- Movement disorder • Parkinsonism • Parkinson disease • Tremor • Dystonia
- Chorea • Tic • Myoclonus

KEY POINTS

- Diagnosis of movement disorders is made clinically, so the neurologic examination is essential.
- The neurologic examination is an extension of the history—a means by which to refine the differential diagnosis and interrogate hypotheses.
- By classifying a movement disorder as hypokinetic or hyperkinetic, the appropriate examination components can be performed to aid in diagnosis.

INTRODUCTION

General practitioners frequently encounter movement disorders in both the inpatient and outpatient settings. Movement disorders can be divided into two broad categories: hypokinetic and hyperkinetic. In the most elementary terms, the former involves loss or slowing of movement, whereas the latter is characterized by excessive and involuntary movements. By determining which category applies to the patient presenting with movement concerns, a narrowed differential is more readily available.

The principal hypokinetic movement disorder is parkinsonism, which includes idiopathic Parkinson disease, Parkinson-plus disorders, and secondary forms of parkinsonism (eg, drug-induced, vascular, etc). Parkinson disease is one of the most common neurologic disorders and is more likely to be diagnosed in older patients, affecting 1% of patients over age 65 years and 2% over age 85 years.[1,2] The hyperkinetic disorders include tremors, choreas, dystonias, tics, and myoclonus. Considering whether the history and physical examination suggest a hypokinetic or hyperkinetic movement disorder can rapidly yield significant clinical insight (**Box 1**).

[a] Department of Neurology, Emory University School of Medicine, 12 Executive Park Drive Northeast, Suite 290, Atlanta, GA 30329, USA; [b] Department of Medicine, Division of General Internal Medicine, Emory University School of Medicine, 49 Jesse Hill Jr. Drive, Atlanta, GA 30303, USA
* Corresponding author.
E-mail address: dwinkel@emory.edu

Med Clin N Am 106 (2022) 519–525
https://doi.org/10.1016/j.mcna.2022.02.002
0025-7125/22/© 2022 Elsevier Inc. All rights reserved.

Box 1	
Initial classification of movement disorders	
Hypokinetic	Idiopathic Parkinson disease
	Parkinson-plus disorders
	Secondary forms of parkinsonism (eg, drug-induced, vascular, etc)
Hyperkinetic	Tremor (eg, physiologic, essential)
	Chorea (eg, Huntington's, Sydenham's)
	Dystonia (eg, genetic, drug-induced)
	Tic (eg, simple motor tics, Tourette's)
	Myoclonus (eg, metabolic, drug-induced, postanoxic)

Definitive diagnosis of movement disorders can only be made either histopathologically (for the neurodegenerative disorders like Parkinson disease) or clinically, and there is no laboratory test or radiologic study that is entirely diagnostic for these disorders. Therefore, in practice, these diagnoses must be made on clinical grounds, using a meticulous history and careful physical examination. The primary care provider is often the first clinician to hear a patient's concerns or discern findings on examination that may suggest a movement disorder. Prompt diagnosis and correct differentiation between movement disorders, made by using screening and focused neurologic examination techniques, can lead to expedient evaluation and appropriate treatments that can improve a patient's quality of life.

NEUROLOGIC EXAMINATION FOR MOVEMENT DISORDERS
Screening Neurologic Examination

The screening neurologic examination should be differential diagnosis-driven and tailored to answer a particular clinical question that emerges from a thoughtful history to uncover neurologic diagnoses that otherwise might be missed. By performing these screening techniques in a primary care setting, more directed physical examination testing can be used and appropriate referrals can be made.

The screening neurologic examination consists of the examination of mental status, cranial nerves, the motor and sensory systems, deep tendon reflexes, coordination, as well as station and gait (**Box 2**).

There are several areas of the screening neurologic examination that can uncover findings concerning for a movement disorder, differentiate between hypokinetic and hyperkinetic movement disorders, or discern these disorders from other neurologic

Box 2
Components of the screening neurologic examination
Mental Status
Cranial Nerves
Motor System
Sensory System
Reflexes
Coordination
Station and Gait

diagnoses. For instance, in a patient presenting with a general concern of "trouble with getting dressed," observation of slowness or stiffness on examination might point to a hypokinetic movement disorder, whereas a tremor with reaching for objects might suggest a hyperkinetic one. It is helpful to ask about *hand dominance*, as there may be subtle asymmetry in strength testing or dexterity in all patients. However, if the dominant hand is in fact the slower one when performing tasks, it may point to a hypokinetic movement disorder.

Assessment of *mental status* is also integral to diagnosing many neurologic diseases and movement disorders are often neurodegenerative. Although motor findings may be the most salient features of these conditions, uncovering issues with mental status or memory may disambiguate the type of movement or other neurologic disorder a patient may have. On the *cranial nerve examination*, when checking extraocular motion, impaired vertical gaze is prominent and found earlier in those with Progressive Supranuclear Palsy (one of the Parkinson-plus syndromes), whereas it is a late finding in idiopathic Parkinson disease. By checking bulk and tone during the *motor examination*, one can differentiate between spasticity and rigidity. Spasticity, caused by pyramidal or upper motor neuron lesions, involves more tone on initiation of movement, worsens with speed, and is often accompanied by weakness, while the rigidity often found in parkinsonian conditions is not velocity-dependent and has a consistent increase in tone throughout the movement.

Movement disorders do not usually include problems discerning sharp from dull *sensation*, decreased *vibratory sense*, or issues with *proprioception*, so any marked abnormality in these examinations or in testing *deep tendon reflexes* should prompt consideration of an alternative or concomitant diagnosis. Examination of *gait* and the *Romberg* test provides insight into several neurologic systems all at once. Abnormal findings on these or the basic coordination examination, such as postural instability, or difficulty initiating or stopping gait, should be further explored with more directed examination of strength and coordination to corroborate a suspected diagnosis of a movement disorder.

Directed Neurologic Examination for Movement Disorders

If and when either the history or the screening neurologic examination raises concern for a movement disorder, a more comprehensive and directed neurologic examination should be performed to clarify the diagnosis.[2] The intent of the advanced examination is to refine the differential diagnosis and explore particular hypotheses generated by the history and screening examination. Patients with parkinsonism often have generalized symptoms such as malaise or fatigue before reporting a tremor, but the most disabling features for those with hypokinetic movement disorders are often slowness, stiffness, difficulty walking, and falls. In contrast, those with hyperkinetic movement disorders will report excessive involuntary movements that interfere with their daily lives. A careful history will guide the examiner to the appropriate category of movement disorders and therefore suggest the additional examination components that will help diagnose and treat the patient's condition.

Hypokinetic movement disorders
The cardinal features of the hypokinetic disorders on the physical examination are akinesia/bradykinesia and rigidity.[3] These are defined as slowness or decreased amplitude in movement, arrests in ongoing movement, and an increase in resistance to passive movement. Three-quarters of patients with Parkinson disease also initially complain of an intermittent resting tremor in their upper extremity that worsens with emotional distress and does not occur with sleep.

The directed neurologic examination begins during the patient interview, with active observation of the patient's *facial expression, general spontaneous movement, and speech*. The hallmarks of a hypokinetic disorder would be diminished facial expression (hypomimia, or "masked facies") and a (fewer blinks than would be expected in a given time period). As opposed to other patients who may, for instance, spontaneously gesture, shift in their seat, or turn their body, patients with hypokinetic movement disorders may exhibit a general paucity of movement. They may also have a shuffling gait or difficulty rising from a chair. In addition, they may have hypophonic, or soft, speech and a "pill-rolling" tremor at rest, in which the index finger flexes and extends against the thumb.

During the confrontational, or hands-on, portion of the examination, one can ask the patient to perform several maneuvers to elicit evidence of movement dysfunction. First, patients can be asked to *tap their index fingers* against their thumbs as quickly and with as high amplitude as they can ("big and fast"). This should be done one side at a time to avoid entraining the faster side to its slower counterpart. Abnormal findings would range from slight slowing of the movement, diminished amplitude of the taps, or pausing during tapping, to barely being able to perform the task due to slowing, interruptions, or decrements in the taps. *Hand clenches* can also be tested, with the patient making a tight fist and then opening and closing the hand repeatedly as fully and as quickly as possible. As before, any slowness, interruptions, or decrement in amplitude are abnormal. Similarly, *heel taps*, in which the physician asks the patient to repetitively strike their heel on the ground, can elicit the same findings for the lower extremities.

Assessment of *rapid alternating movements* is another important technique to help in diagnosing hypokinetic movement disorders. The patient begins by resting one hand on their thigh, palmar aspect down, subsequently turning it over into a supinated position, and strikes it back down so that the dorsal aspect strikes the thigh. The hand should then be turned back over so that the palmar aspect strikes the thigh; this should be repeated several times, with pronation and supination alternating as quickly and decisively as possible. As before, each side should be tested independently. Abnormalities range from slight slowing or interruption of the cadence of the rapid alternating movements to repeated interruptions, significant slowing, or even a prolonged arrest of the task.

Gait should be examined as well, with the patient asked to walk away from and toward the examiner so that both sides of the body can be easily observed simultaneously. Gait abnormalities associated with hypokinetic movement disorders include difficulty initiating gait, slowness, stooped posture, decreased arm swing, and "freezing," or an arrest of gait, often noted while stepping through doorways.

Examination of muscle *tone* is another important diagnostic aspect of the directed examination. This is best done with the examiner passively moving a patient's completely relaxed limb in a variety of directions to evaluate the intrinsic resistance of the limb. To relax one side, the patient can be asked to perform a cognitive task with the other limb as a form of distraction, such as tapping fingers while they count down from 10. A finding of rigidity, an increase in the limb's resistance to passive movement, is abnormal. The so-called cogwheel rigidity, a ratchet-like intermittent resistance during passive movement of a limb, is one of the cardinal features of parkinsonism (**Box 3**).

Patients with parkinsonism will often have been initiated on carbidopa-levodopa before a subsequent primary care visit. In those cases, it is recommended one ask the patient to arrive without taking their carbidopa-levodopa and then take it at the onset of the session. The rapid onset of the drug allows the patient to be examined

Box 3
Components of the Directed neurologic examination for hypokinetic movement disorders
Facial expression
General spontaneous movement
Speech
Finger taps
Hand clenches
Heel taps
Rapid alternating movements
Gait
Muscle Tone

"off" and then "on" the drug, with direct comparison of the aforementioned directed neurologic examination techniques. This strategy can help the provider clarify whether or not the patient is responding to the drug and dose.

Hyperkinetic movement disorders

Tremors, choreas, dystonias, tic, and myoclonus comprise most hyperkinetic movement disorders.[4] From the perspective of the diagnostician, careful observation of the patient's movements and postures is often more illuminating than performance of the confrontational examination, which may, in fact, interfere with and obscure the movements of interest.

Tremors are involuntary rhythmic shaking movements involving one or more body parts. The pattern, distribution, and clinical characteristics of tremors can help clarify their etiology. Tremor types include resting (occurring while the limb is at rest), postural (occurring while the limb is held to maintain posture against gravity), or kinetic (occurring during a goal-directed movement). To distinguish these, the patient may be observed with their limbs at rest (eg, placed upon their lap), while holding each limb aloft in an outstretched manner, and while purposefully reaching toward a target (eg, reaching to touch the examiner's finger). These simple examination techniques can help differentiate the etiology of a patient's tremors. For instance, parkinsonian tremors are easily seen with the patient resting their hands in their lap and are slow in frequency, while essential, familial, tremors are bilateral and exacerbated with maintaining posture against gravity or with targeted movement.

Dystonias are abnormal postures and involuntary, sustained muscle contractions that produce twisting or squeezing movements and are best simply observed. These contractions may be complicated by repetitive movements that vary in speed, and that may result in fixed postures resulting from the sustained muscle contractions. These contractions are typically stereotyped, meaning that the assumed posture or movement looks similar each time it occurs. Interestingly, patients are often aware of a means through which they can temporarily relax the muscle contraction to relieve the dystonia, a phenomenon referred to as a "sensory trick."

Choreas are excessive, spontaneous movements, often with a dance-like quality that involves multiple body parts. They are irregularly timed, nonrepetitive, and randomly distributed. They can either be diffuse and symmetric, or restricted to a single side of the body, termed hemichorea.

Tics are repetitive, brief, rapid, involuntary, purposeless, stereotyped movements that involve single or multiple muscle groups. Motor tics are often accompanied by vocal tics

---

Box 4
Directed neurologic examination for hyperkinetic movement disorders

Observation of quality and character of movement

Evaluate tremor at rest, with posture, and during movement

Inquire about "sensory trick" if dystonia suspected

---

which, most often, are grunts and other rudimentary vocalizations, but rarely, as in Tourette syndrome, may involve verbal tics composed of obscenities. Motor tics are classically associated with an intense and escalating urge to tic, with relief immediately following the tic. With significant effort, they may also be temporarily suppressible.

Myoclonus is a rapid, shock-like, arrhythmic, and often repetitive set of involuntary movements. These movements may be focal, multifocal, or generalized (**Box 4**).

REFERRAL VERSUS REASSURANCE

In general, conditions that appear at significant risk of rapid progression and subsequent harm to the patient should be promptly referred to a Neurologist. With regards to the movement disorders, the signs and symptoms of concern (the "red flags") include frequent falls, unilateral symptoms, abrupt onset or rapid progression, associated cranial nerve palsies, impairment of activities of daily living, and weakness or muscle wasting. In contrast, relatively reassuring signs and symptoms include mild nonbothersome or symmetric symptoms and lack of progression of symptoms over time. This is not to imply that patients lacking "red flags" would not ultimately benefit from neurologic consultation, but there is likely no urgency to the referral. For instance, a patient describing a mild, nonbothersome, intermittent, postural tremor symmetrically involving both hands that has been present for several years and does not interfere with any activities the patient wishes to engage in likely requires nothing more than reassurance. In contrast, a patient with progression of bradykinesia or rigidity over the past few months, now culminating in weekly falls, should be promptly referred.

SUMMARY

Movement disorders are commonly encountered by the primary care physician, both in the ambulatory and inpatient settings. A careful history, observation, and performance of the screening and more directed neurologic examinations are essential in diagnosing movement disorders as there are no laboratory findings or other studies that are diagnostic. Categorizing a movement disorder as hypokinetic versus hyperkinetic, or characterized by slowness, stiffness, and loss of movement versus by excessive, involuntary movement will narrow the differential and lead to expedient treatment and referral, if needed. Neurologic consultation should be considered for both rapid diagnosis and long-term management of movement disorders and should be expedited in the case of any "red flags" on the history or physical examination.

CLINICS CARE POINTS

- A nuanced and comprehensive history will generate a focused differential diagnosis for movement disorders
- The screening and directed neurologic examinations help refine the clinician's differential diagnosis for movement disorders and interrogate hypotheses

- It can be very helpful to classify a movement disorder as hypokinetic or hyperkinetic
- Patients with frequent falls, unilateral symptoms, abrupt onset or rapid progression, associated cranial nerve palsies, impairment of activities of daily living, and weakness or muscle wasting should be promptly referred to a Neurologist

DISCLOSURE

The authors have nothing to disclose.

REFERENCES

1. Ben-Shlomo Y. The epidemiology of Parkinson's disease. Baillieres Clin Neurol 1997;6(1):55–68.
2. Simel DL, Drummond R. Parkinsonism." *The rational clinical examination: evidence-based clinical diagnosis*. McGraw Hill; 2009. Available at: https://jamaevidence-mhmedical-com.proxy.library.emory.edu/content.aspx?bookid=845&sectionid=61357583.
3. Olanow C, Klein C, Schapira AV. Parkinson's disease. In: Jameson J, Fauci AS, Kasper DL, et al, editors. Harrison's principles of internal medicine, 20nd edition. McGraw Hill; 2018.
4. Olanow C, Klein C, Obeso JA. Tremor, chorea, and other movement disorders. In: Jameson J, Fauci AS, Kasper DL, et al, editors. Harrison's principles of internal medicine, 20nd edition. McGraw Hill; 2018.

Physical Examination in Human Immunodeficiency Virus Disease

Christopher L. Knight, MD

KEYWORDS

- Physical examination • HIV • AIDS • Kaposi sarcoma • Bacillary angiomatosis
- Oral hairy leukoplakia

KEY POINTS

- HIV has many manifestations that appear on physical examination.
- Findings in HIV are often caused by a combination of HIV itself and associated opportunistic infections.
- Many findings in HIV disease become more prevalent or more dramatic as the disease progresses.
- The skin and oropharynx are especially rich sources of HIV-associated findings.
- Although there is no single finding that is diagnostic of HIV disease, a constellation of findings in the appropriate clinical setting should make one strongly suspect HIV infection.

INTRODUCTION

Human immunodeficiency virus (HIV)-associated disease is known for its protean manifestations. However, in the case of HIV, many of the characteristic findings on physical examination are not associated with HIV infection per se but the numerous opportunistic infections (OIs) that are common in patients with advanced HIV disease. The goal of this article is to outline both the manifestations of HIV itself and some of the typical findings of common OIs. In observing both facets of HIV's presentation, the skilled clinician can identify likely HIV infection in both early and late stages of the disease.

PRIMARY HUMAN IMMUNODEFICIENCY VIRUS AND COMPLICATIONS OF THERAPY

Acute Human Immunodeficiency Virus Infection

Initial HIV infection typically presents as an acute viral syndrome within 2 to 6 weeks of acquisition of the disease.[1] The most common presenting symptom or sign is fever, present in more than 90% of patients with acute HIV infection.[2] Other common

University of Washington, 1959 NE Pacific St, Seattle, WA 98195, USA
E-mail address: cknight@uw.edu
Twitter: @clknight (C.L.K.)

Med Clin N Am 106 (2022) 527–536
https://doi.org/10.1016/j.mcna.2022.01.001
0025-7125/22/© 2022 Elsevier Inc. All rights reserved.

findings include adenopathy (50%–90% of patients),[2,3] rash (35%–77% of patients),[2,4] and oral ulcers (30%–35%).[3,4]

Early HIV infection can also present with an aseptic meningitis-like syndrome, with fever, headache, photophobia, and stiff neck. Some patients have elevated cerebrospinal fluid leukocyte counts, although the absolute number of leukocytes tends to be low (<10).[2]

Chronic Human Immunodeficiency Virus Disease

Although many findings in chronic HIV disease are associated with OIs, there are several skin findings associated with advanced disease that have not yet been demonstrated to be infectious in cause. These findings include eosinophilic folliculitis,[5] characterized by 3- to 5-mm urticarial follicular papules on the trunk, head, and neck that are intensely pruritic. Eosinophilia is present on biopsy and sometimes also in peripheral blood. Eosinophilic folliculitis is typically seen when CD4 counts decrease to less than 250/mm³. The cornerstone of therapy is treatment of HIV; lesions typically resolve as the CD4 count climbs, although they can initially worsen with immune reconstitution.[6] Clubbing of the nails has also been observed in chronic HIV disease (**Fig. 1**). One report found it in 36% of patients with HIV, in the absence of other causes of clubbing.[7] HIV disease is also associated with increased severity of other dermatologic conditions, including psoriasis and drug eruptions.

HIV can have several rheumatologic manifestations.[8] Patients with HIV have higher rates of reactive arthritis (typically with more dramatic skin involvement) and spondyloarthropathies. Those with psoriatic arthritis may have more severe joint disease along with worsened cutaneous psoriasis. HIV can also cause a primary arthropathy that can present with an asymmetric oligoarthritis typically involving knees/ankles, or a symmetric polyarthritis similar to rheumatoid arthritis.

Neurologic findings can also occur in chronic HIV disease. Distal sensory polyneuropathy is common, affecting as many as 35% of patients with advanced disease, and can cause decreased sensation of vibration, pain, and temperature as well as diminished ankle reflexes.[9] Neuropathy is also thought to be a common complication of antiretroviral therapy, although some evidence suggests that appropriate treatment may improve symptoms in patients with neuropathy.[10,11]

Complications

In addition to neuropathy, antiretroviral therapy for HIV can cause a variety of adverse effects, most of which lack specific physical findings.[12] One notable exception is

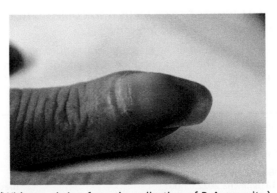

Fig. 1. Clubbing. (With permission from the collection of P. Aronowitz.)

lipodystrophy, which has been noted with both nucleoside reverse transcriptase inhibitors and protease inhibitors. Patients with lipodystrophy frequently have both accumulation of central fat in the trunk and atrophy of peripheral fat in the extremities and face, leading to a characteristic pattern of changes in appearance.[13] Lipodystrophy is associated with metabolic disease and increased cardiovascular risk.[14]

OPPORTUNISTIC INFECTIONS
Seborrheic Dermatitis

Seborrheic dermatitis is a common skin disorder that presents with scale and erythema of the scalp and face. Patients with pigmented skin may also have hypopigmentation in areas of seborrheic dermatitis, and postlesional hyperpigmentation is common.[15] The condition is associated with *Malassezia* yeast species, although its role in pathogenesis is complex and multifactorial. Seborrheic dermatitis is both more prevalent and more severe in patients with HIV than in the general population. Prevalence estimates range from 20% to 83%, and the scale in patients with HIV is often thicker and heavier, sometimes occurring in atypical locations.[16]

Scabies

Patients with advanced HIV disease are at increased risk of a severe form of scabies infection called crusted or Norwegian scabies (**Fig. 2**). Crusted scabies manifests as hyperkeratotic plaques with cracking and scaling and can mimic psoriasis or severe seborrheic dermatitis.[17] The mite burden in patients with crusted scabies is very high, and nosocomial transmission has been reported when inadequate isolation measures are used.[17,18]

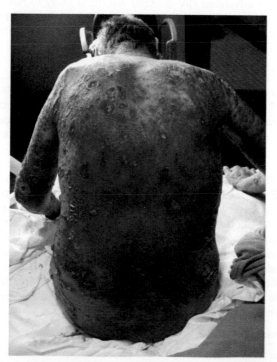

Fig. 2. Crusted scabies. (With permission from the collection of P. Aronowitz.)

Herpes Simplex

Herpes simplex virus (HSV) coinfection is extremely common with HIV, with 70% seropositive for HSV-2 and an additional 25% seropositive for HSV-1 or both.[19] Clinical manifestations of HSV in patients with HIV include typical genital and orolabial lesions but can also cause severe, extensive ulcerations in patients with low CD4 counts.[20] Rarely, HSV can cause hypertrophic lesions mimicking neoplasia.[21]

Herpes Zoster

Reactivation of varicella zoster virus (VZV) infection is extremely common among patients with HIV and high levels of immunosuppression, occurring at 15-fold higher rates than the general population.[19] The cutaneous manifestations of herpes zoster in most patients with HIV are similar to those of immunocompetent patients: a painful vesicular eruption in a dermatomal distribution, often with a prodrome of pain or numbness before the rash appears. However, patients with CD4 counts less than 200 cells/mm^3 are also at higher risk of multidermatomal and disseminated herpes zoster infections.[22] Multidermatomal zoster can present without the typical distribution of the rash, and disseminated zoster can also have central nervous system manifestations including vasculitis, myelitis, and encephalitis. Treatment of HIV reduces the risk of severe VZV reactivation and the accompanying complications, although there is an increased risk of reactivation of VZV in the first 3 months after initiating antiretroviral therapy.[19]

Molluscum Contagiosum

Molluscum contagiosum is a common viral infection caused by a member of the poxvirus family. In immunocompetent patients, molluscum manifests as small umbilicated lesions averaging 3 to 5 mm in diameter and typically limited to 20 lesions or fewer. Patients with advanced HIV disease are more likely to have larger numbers of lesions and atypical locations including the face. Lesions may also be atypical in appearance, lacking central umbilication or coalescing into "giant" molluscum lesions greater than 1 cm in diameter.[23]

Human Papilloma Virus

Human papilloma virus (HPV) is a common cause of both genital/cutaneous warts and skin and mucosal cancers. Patients with HIV are at increased risk of both.[19] Genital and cutaneous warts in patients with HIV are usually of typical appearance but may be larger or more extensive than in a nonimmunosuppressed patient.

Kaposi Sarcoma

Kaposi sarcoma (KS) is a vascular neoplasm associated with human herpesvirus 8, also known as KS-associated herpesvirus. The most common site for KS involvement is the skin, where KS lesions usually start as flat lesions and then become more nodular or plaquelike as the tumor enlarges. The color varies because of the vascular nature of the lesion: they can be pink, red, brown, or purple, but they are usually palpable and nonpruritic[24] (**Fig. 3**). Visceral KS lesions may bleed, presenting with hematemesis, melena, hematochezia, or hemoptysis. Oral lesions in patients with untreated HIV may be associated with increased mortality risk.[25] Although antineoplastic therapy for KS is available, successful treatment of HIV is frequently sufficient to resolve KS lesions in many patients.[26]

Bacillary Angiomatosis

Bacillary angiomatosis refers to nodular, angioproliferative skin lesions caused by infection by Bartonella bacteria. Lesions are typically nodules and plaques, ranging

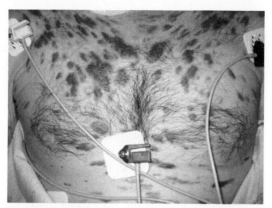

Fig. 3. Kaposi sarcoma. (With permission from the collection of P. Aronowitz.)

from pink to brown-red depending on underlying skin pigmentation (**Fig. 4**). Lesions are usually more friable than KS lesions and often bleed easily on contact, sometimes mimicking pyogenic granuloma.[15,27] Definitive diagnosis depends on demonstrating the organism in tissue, either histologically or using tissue polymerase chain reaction testing. Therapy should include antimicrobials directed at *Bartonella* in addition to treatment of HIV disease.[24]

OROPHARYNGEAL
Candidiasis

Oropharygeal candidiasis is common among people with HIV and is a marker for immune suppression, occurring more often in patients with low CD4 counts.[28] The most common form is pseudomembranous candidiasis (thrush), consisting of white plaques that adhere to oral mucosal surfaces, including the tongue, palate, gums, and buccal mucosa (**Fig. 5**). However, *Candida* infection may also present as an atrophic or erythematous form, consisting of flat, red erythematous lesions on the palate or tongue, or as angular cheilitis, with cracking and erythema at the corners of the mouth.[24] Disease-specific treatment consists of topical or systemic antifungal therapy. Treatment of HIV with highly active antiretroviral therapy (HAART) is associated with a reduced risk of all forms of oral candidiasis.[29]

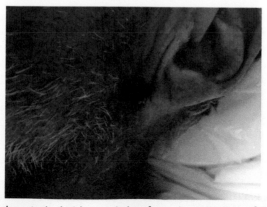

Fig. 4. Bacillary angiomatosis. (With permission from the collection of P. Aronowitz.)

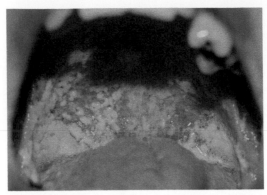

Fig. 5. Oropharyngeal candidiasis. (*Photograph from* David Spach, MD, reproduced with permission National HIV Curriculum.)

Hairy Leukoplakia

Oral hairy leukoplakia (OHL) is a physical finding strongly associated with moderate to severe immunosuppression in patients with HIV.[30] OHL is characterized by raised white lesions, typically on the lateral aspects of the tongue but sometimes involving buccal and pharyngeal mucosa (**Fig. 6**). OHL lesions are adherent to the underlying mucosa and cannot be easily removed with a tongue blade, which helps to distinguish them from candidiasis.[31] Epstein-Barr virus is strongly associated with the lesions, although the precise mechanism of pathogenesis is unclear. Treatment of HIV will usually lead to resolution of OHL lesions.[24]

Other

HSV, HPV, and KS can all cause oropharyngeal lesions that are similar to their cutaneous manifestations noted earlier. As with cutaneous disease, oral manifestations of HSV and HPV are often more extensive or more severe in patients with advanced immunosuppression. Treatment of HIV with HAART can be curative for KS and reduce severity and frequency of HSV lesions, but does not seem to improve warts and may even increase prevalence based on one study.[32]

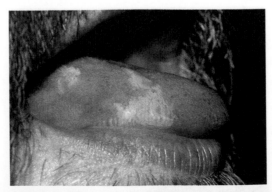

Fig. 6. Oral hairy leukoplakia. (*Photograph from* David Spach, MD, reproduced with permission National HIV Curriculum.)

OCULAR
Herpes Zoster Ophthalmicus

Reactivation of varicella-zoster virus (VZV) involving the ophthalmic branch of the trigeminal nerve can result in herpes zoster ophthalmicus (HZO); this can manifest as corneal inflammation (keratitis), anterior uveitis, or retinal necrosis. Patients with VZV keratitis often have corneal ulceration with a dendritic pattern.[33] Patients with VZV uveitis have eye pain and photophobia, whereas those with retinitis may present with visual loss and evidence of retinal injury or retinal detachment on funduscopic examination. One clue to ocular involvement with VZV is the presence of vesicular lesions on the tip of the nose (Hutchinson sign), which reflects involvement of the nasociliary branch of the ophthalmic nerve. However, this finding is present in only 22% of patients with HZO.[34]

Cytomegalovirus Retinitis

Cytomegalovirus (CMV) is a member of the herpesvirus family that causes multisystem disease in immunosuppressed patients. CMV retinitis is the ophthalmic manifestation of CMV infection and is most prevalent in patients with HIV and advanced immunosuppression (CD4 count < 50/mm^3).[35] Funduscopic examination in patients with CMV retinitis shows fluffy, yellow-white lesions with tiny "satellite" lesions at the border with normal retina; hemorrhage may or may not be present.[19] Treatment of CMV retinitis includes disease-specific antiviral therapy (usually ganciclovir) combined with treatment of HIV in those not already on antiretroviral therapy.[19] Because immune reconstitution can precipitate uveitis, patients should be watched closely when initiating antiretroviral therapy.

NEUROLOGIC
Toxoplasma Encephalitis

Toxoplasmosis is a parasitic infection that most often manifests in patients with HIV who have a CD4 count less than 100/mm^3.[24] The most common site of infection is the brain, and patients frequently present with fever, confusion, and headache. Focal neurologic findings were present in 69% of patients in a large case series, most frequently hemiparesis, ataxia, and cranial nerve deficits.[36] Treatment of toxoplasma encephalitis includes antiparasitic therapy and treatment of HIV in those not already on antiretroviral therapy.[19]

Cryptococcal Meningitis

Cryptococcal infection in patients with HIV usually causes a subacute meningitis with fever, malaise, and headache evolving over weeks. Almost 90% of patients have a CD4 count less than 100/mm^3.[24] Physical examination findings are notably nonspecific: in one case series only 48% of patients had any focal deficit on neurologic examination and only 37% had a stiff neck. Initial therapy is with antifungal agents alone; cryptococcal meningitis is one of the few OIs in which initiating antiretroviral therapy early results in worse outcomes.[19]

Progressive Multifocal Leukoencephalopathy

The JC virus is a common polyoma virus, named after the initials of the first patient from whom it was isolated. In people with a normal immune system the virus remains latent. In those with severe immunosuppression, including advanced HIV disease, it can reactivate and infect glial cells in the central nervous system, causing the demyelinating disease progressive multifocal leukoencephalopathy (PML).[37] The clinical course of PML is characterized by gradually worsening focal neurologic deficits. Specific examination findings vary based on the anatomic location of the white matter lesions; one cohort study found that the most common presenting symptoms were impaired coordination, cognitive defects, speech disturbance, limb paresis, and visual impairment.[38] There is no disease-specific therapy, and treatment of the underlying HIV disease is the cornerstone of management.

SUMMARY

HIV is a famously protean disease. Primary HIV infection mimics other viral syndromes, whereas late-stage HIV disease can present with a panoply of abnormalities related to multiple OIs. However, when an astute clinician recognizes that a constellation of findings is suggestive of HIV disease and makes the diagnosis, it can open the door to highly effective, lifesaving therapies.

CLINICS CARE POINTS

- Acute HIV manifests similarly to other viral syndromes. Clinicians should have a low threshold for testing in patients with risk factors for exposure.
- Antiretroviral therapy can cause some of the common findings in HIV, including lipodystrophy and neuropathy.
- Skin manifestations of HIV are extremely frequent and include both exacerbations of common infections (seborrheic dermatitis, scabies, HSV, VZV, molluscum, HPV) and rare conditions associated with immunosuppression (KS, bacillary angiomatosis)
- Patients may have oral candidiasis without the typical adherent plaques of thrush.
- Oral hairy leukoplakia can be distinguished from *Candida* by inability to scrape it off with a tongue blade.
- The presence of zoster lesions on the tip of the nose (Hutchinson sign) is suggestive of ophthalmic involvement.
- Cryptococcal meningitis is one of the few infections in which one waits to initiate antiviral therapy for HIV.

DISCLOSURE

The author has nothing to disclose.

REFERENCES

1. Quinn TC. Acute primary HIV infection. JAMA 1997;278(1):58–62.
2. Schacker T, Collier AC, Hughes J, et al. Clinical and epidemiologic features of primary HIV infection. Ann Intern Med 1996;125(4):257.
3. Gaines H, Sydow M von, Pehrson PO, et al. Clinical picture of primary HIV infection presenting as a glandular-fever-like illness. BMJ 1988;297(6660):1363.
4. Lapins J, Gaines H, Lindbä S, et al. Skin and mucosal characteristics of symptomatic primary HIV-1 infection. AIDS Patient Care STDS 1997;11(2):67–70.
5. Rosenthal D, LeBoit PE, Klumpp L, et al. Human Immunodeficiency virus-associated eosinophilic folliculitis: a unique dermatosis associated with advanced human immunodeficiency virus infection. Arch Dermatol 1991;127(2):206–9.

6. Fearfield Rowe, Francis Bunker. Staughton. Itchy folliculitis and human immuno-deficiency virus infection: clinicopathological and immunological features, patho-genesis and treatment. Br J Dermatol 1999;141(1):3–11.

7. Dever LL, Matta JS. Digital clubbing in HIV-infected patients: an observational study. Aids Patient Care St 2009;23(1):19–22.

8. Adizie T, Moots RJ, Hodkinson B, et al. Inflammatory arthritis in HIV positive pa-tients: a practical guide. BMC Infect Dis 2016;16(1):100.

9. Schifitto G, McDermott MP, McArthur JC, et al. Incidence of and risk factors for HIV-associated distal sensory polyneuropathy. Neurology 2002;58(12):1764–8.

10. Centner CM, Little F, Watt JJ, et al. Evolution of sensory neuropathy after initiation of antiretroviral therapy. Muscle Nerve 2018;57(3):371–9.

11. Kaku M, Simpson DM. HIV, antiretrovirals, and peripheral neuropathy: a moving target. Muscle Nerve 2018;57(3):347–9.

12. Margolis AM, Heverling H, Pham PA, et al. A review of the toxicity of HIV medica-tions. J Med Toxicol 2014;10(1):26–39.

13. Mallon P, Cooper D, Carr A. HIV-associated lipodystrophy. Hiv Med 2001;2(3): 166–73.

14. Grinspoon S, Carr A. Cardiovascular risk and body-fat abnormalities in HIV-infected adults. N Engl J Med 2005;352(1):48–62.

15. Motswaledi MH, Visser W. The spectrum of HIV-associated infective and inflam-matory dermatoses in pigmented skin. Dermatol Clin 2014;32(2):211–25.

16. Adalsteinsson JA, Kaushik S, Muzumdar S, et al. An update on the microbiology, immunology and genetics of seborrheic dermatitis. Exp Dermatol 2020;29(5): 481–9.

17. Heukelbach J, Feldmeier H. Scabies. Lancet 2006;367(9524):1767–74.

18. Corbett EL, Crossley I, Holton J, et al. Crusted ("Norwegian") scabies in a specialist HIV unit: successful use of ivermectin and failure to prevent nosocomial transmission. Genitourin Med 1996;72(2):115.

19. HIV. P on G for the P and T of OI in A and A with. Guidelines for the Prevention and Treatment of Opportunistic Infections in HIV-infected Adults and Adolescents: Recommendations from the Centers for Disease Control and Prevention, the Na-tional Institutes of Health, and the HIV Medicine Association of the Infectious Dis-eases Society of America. Available at: https://clinicalinfo.hiv.gov/sites/default/files/inline-files/adult_oi.pdf. Accessed October 29, 2021.

20. Strick LB, Wald A, Celum C. Management of herpes simplex virus type 2 infection in HIV type 1–infected persons. Clin Infect Dis 2006;43(3):347–56.

21. Sbidian E, Battistella M, LeGoff J, et al. Recalcitrant pseudotumoral anogenital herpes simplex virus type 2 in HIV-infected patients: evidence for predominant B-lymphoplasmocytic infiltration and immunomodulators as effective therapeutic strategy. Clin Infect Dis 2013;57(11):1648–55.

22. Veenstra J, van Praag RME, Krol A, et al. Complications of varicella zoster virus reactivation in HIV-infected homosexual men. Aids 1996;10(4):393–400.

23. Meza-Romero R, Navarrete-Dechent C, Downey C. Molluscum contagiosum: an update and review of new perspectives in etiology, diagnosis, and treatment. Clin Cosmet Investig Dermatol 2019;12:373–81.

24. Spach DH. National HIV curriculum: cutaneous manifestations. Accessed. https://www.hiv.uw.edu/go/basic-primary-care/cutaneous-manifestations/core-concept/all. [Accessed 29 October 2021]. Avaiable at.

25. Rohrmus B, Thoma-Greber EM, Bogner JR, et al. Outlook in oral and cutaneous Kaposi's sarcoma. Lancet 2000;356(9248):2160.

26. Bower M, Weir J, Francis N, et al. The effect of HAART in 254 consecutive patients with AIDS-related Kaposi's sarcoma. Aids 2009;23(13):1701–6.
27. Cotell SL, Noskin GA. Bacillary angiomatosis. Clinical and histologic features, diagnosis, and treatment. Arch Intern Med 1994;154(5):524–8.
28. Ottria L, Lauritano D, Oberti L, et al. Prevalence of HIV-related oral manifestations and their association with HAART and CD4+ T cell count: a review. J Biol Regul Homeost Agents 2018;32(2 Suppl. 1):51–9.
29. Almeida VL de, Lima IFP, Ziegelmann PK, et al. Impact of highly active antiretroviral therapy on the prevalence of oral lesions in HIV-positive patients: a systematic review and meta-analysis. Int J Oral Maxillofac Surg 2017;46(11):1497–504.
30. Husak R, Garbe C, Orfanos CE. Oral hairy leukoplakia in 71 HIV-seropositive patients: Clinical symptoms, relation to immunologic status, and prognostic significance. J Am Acad Dermatol 1996;35(6):928–34.
31. Triantos D, Porter SR, Scully C, et al. Oral hairy leukoplakia: clinicopathologic features, pathogenesis, diagnosis, and clinical significance. Clin Infect Dis 1997; 25(6):1392–6.
32. Greenspan D, Canchola AJ, MacPhail LA, et al. Effect of highly active antiretroviral therapy on frequency of oral warts. Lancet 2001;357(9266):1411–2.
33. Li JY. Herpes zoster ophthalmicus. Curr Opin Ophthalmol 2018;29(4):328–33.
34. Szeto SKH, Chan TCY, Wong RLM, et al. Prevalence of ocular manifestations and visual outcomes in patients with herpes zoster ophthalmicus. Cornea 2017;36(3): 338–42.
35. Kuppermann BD, Petty JG, Richman DD, et al. Correlation between CD4+ counts and prevalence of cytomegalovirus retinitis and human immunodeficiency virus–related noninfectious retinal vasculopathy in patients with acquired immunodeficiency syndrome. Am J Ophthalmol 1993;115(5):575–82.
36. Porter SB, Sande MA. Toxoplasmosis of the central nervous system in the acquired immunodeficiency syndrome. New Engl J Med 1992;327(23):1643–8.
37. Ferenczy MW, Marshall LJ, Nelson CDS, et al. Molecular biology, epidemiology, and pathogenesis of progressive multifocal leukoencephalopathy, the JC virus-induced demyelinating disease of the human brain. Clin Microbiol Rev 2012; 25(3):471–506.
38. Engsig FN, Hansen ABE, Omland LH, et al. Incidence, clinical presentation, and outcome of progressive multifocal leukoencephalopathy in HIV-infected patients during the highly active antiretroviral therapy era: a nationwide cohort study. J Infect Dis 2009;199(1):77–83.

Can't Miss Infections
Endocarditis, Cellulitis, Erysipelas, Necrotizing Fasciitis, Cholecystitis

Kim Tartaglia, MD

KEYWORDS

- Skin and soft tissue infections • Cellulitis • Erysipelas • Necrotizing fasciitis
- Cholecystitis • Infective endocarditis

KEY POINTS

- In cellulitis and erysipelas, the diagnosis is made by history and physical examination. For necrotizing fasciitis, the physical examination is suggestive and the diagnosis is made with the aid of adjunctive laboratory and radiologic testing.
- The physical examination of endocarditis most commonly includes fever and a cardiac murmur. Diagnosis requires additional microbiologic and imaging criteria and the use of the modified Duke Criteria is helpful in making a diagnosis of endocarditis.
- In acute cholecystitis, the physical examination is supportive but diagnosis requires imaging by ultrasound. The physical examination may be less sensitive in the elderly in which tenderness may be absent.

CELLULITIS, ERYSIPELAS, AND NECROTIZING FASCIITIS

Skin and soft tissue infections are common and can be divided into nonpurulent and purulent infections. This review will include common and severe nonpurulent skin infections, including cellulitis, erysipelas, and necrotizing fasciitis.

Cellulitis is a bacterial infection of the deep dermis and may extend into the subcutaneous tissues. Unlike in abscesses, culture data are rarely helpful in determining the underlying etiology of cellulitis. When bacterial data are obtained, concentrations of bacterial growth are low, suggesting that either bacterial toxins and/or inflammatory mediators are responsible for much of the signs and symptoms.[1] Gram-positive skin flora, including group A streptococcus and less commonly staphylococcus aureus, are frequent causative agents.[2] Risk factors for cellulitis include lymphedema, superficial fungal infections, or anything that disrupts the integrity of the skin barrier.[1,2]

Erysipelas (**Fig. 1**, erysipelas of the lower extremity, with permission from the collection of P. Aronowitz) is a superficial dermal skin infection that has marked erythema

Department of Internal Medicine, The Ohio State University College of Medicine, M112 Starling Loving Hall, 310 W 10th Avenue, Columbus, OH 43210, USA
E-mail address: Kimberly.tartaglia@osumc.edu
Twitter: @KimTartaglia (K.T.)

Med Clin N Am 106 (2022) 537–543
https://doi.org/10.1016/j.mcna.2021.12.008
0025-7125/22/© 2022 Elsevier Inc. All rights reserved.

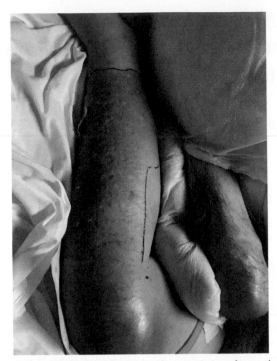

Fig. 1. Erysipelas of the lower extremity. (*with permission* from the collection of P. Aronowitz)

and well-demarcated raised borders. It commonly occurs on the lower extremities or face and *Streptococcus pyogenes* is the usual bacterial cause. It often starts at a disruption in the skin from trauma or on the feet or between the toes from tinea pedis (**Fig. 2**, tinea pedis in a patient with erysipelas, with permission from the collection of P. Aronowitz) infection and travels via the lymphatic system. It is this lymphatic involvement in the lower extremities that often explains the presence of acute, tender inguinal lymphadenopathy proximal to the affected leg. The physical examination should therefore include a careful search for a portal of entry in the skin as well as for the presence of inguinal adenopathy.

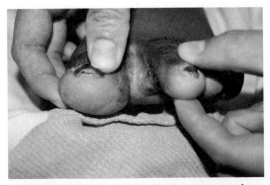

Fig. 2. Tinea pedis in a patient with erysipelas. (*with permission* from the collection of P. Aronowitz)

The diagnosis of cellulitis and erysipelas is made by history and physical examination. Physical examination in cellulitis commonly reveals poorly demarcated, spreading erythema, warmth, and tenderness. Fever is variably present, ranging from 20% to 70% of the time when assessed in the emergency department and inpatient settings.[1,2] For patients with localized cellulitis, careful examination should assess for the presence of a deeper abscess. Ultrasound examination can be useful in evaluating for abscess if the bedside examination is not definitive.

The differential diagnosis for cellulitis includes stasis dermatitis, deep vein thrombosis, and hematoma that may have been induced by trauma or anticoagulation.[1] Stasis dermatitis is most often bilateral and cellulitis is almost always unilateral. Deep vein thrombosis is an uncommon comorbid condition in cellulitis and was only found in the ipsilateral leg at a rate of 0.75%.[3] If erythema is overlying a joint, gout is a consideration that is commonly confused with cellulitis. Less commonly, erythema migrans or calciphylaxis is confused for cellulitis.[1,2]

Treatment of cellulitis includes systemic antimicrobial therapy. Antimicrobial therapy targeted to most likely agents is recommended and treatment duration is generally 5 days, although can be extended in special circumstances.[2]

Necrotizing fasciitis is a severe, rapidly progressive infection of the subcutaneous tissues and fascia that is associated with high mortality and requires urgent identification and surgical referral. Causative agents include gram-positives and mixed aerobic-anaerobic bacteria. Empiric broad-spectrum antibiotics are recommended initially to cover both staphylococcus aureus and anaerobes.[2,4]

The physical examination in necrotizing fasciitis is associated with tenderness out of proportion to the examination. Clinical findings may include edema, necrosis, crepitus, and cutaneous numbness.

The diagnosis of necrotizing fasciitis is made by clinical examination with support from laboratory and radiologic evidence. In necrotizing fasciitis, the white blood cell count and inflammatory markers are typically elevated. Additionally, the laboratory risk index for necrotizing fasciitis (LRINEC) developed by Wong, and colleagues uses white blood cell count, C-reactive protein, hemoglobin, serum sodium, serum creatinine, and serum glucose to develop a risk calculation for necrotizing fasciitis.[4,5] Initial studies suggested a sensitivity of 90% with a positive likelihood ratio of 19.95 and a negative likelihood ratio of 0.10.[5] Computed tomography is an adjunctive test to diagnosing necrotizing fasciitis and has a negative predictive value of 100%.[4]

INFECTIVE ENDOCARDITIS

Infective endocarditis refers to an infection of the endocardial surface of the heart and typically involves infection of the heart valves. Risk factors for infective endocarditis include history of congenital heart or valve disease, nonnative valves or other material in the heart, intravenous drug use, and recent dental or surgical procedures.[6]

The presenting signs and symptoms of endocarditis vary based on whether the infection is acute or subacute. Symptoms are often nonspecific with the most common symptom being fever in up to 90% of patients.[6,7] Other symptoms can include night sweats, anorexia, weight loss, myalgias, joint pain, and fatigue. The physical examination demonstrates a cardiac murmur in 85% of patients.[7] Extracardiac manifestations are less common but may include splenomegaly and cutaneous signs, such as splinter hemorrhages (**Fig. 3**, from the collection of P. Aronowitz), clubbing (**Fig. 4**, from the collection of P. Aronowitz), Janeway lesions, Osler nodes (**Fig. 5**, with permission from the collection of T. Levy) and petechiae. Additional presenting clinical manifestations may occur as a result of septic emboli or systemic immune reaction; these

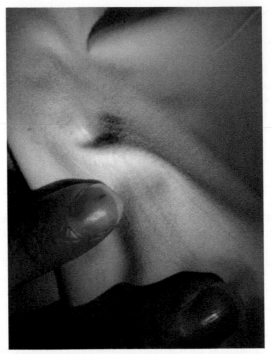

Fig. 3. Clubbing. (*from* the collection of P. Aronowitz)

manifestations include stroke, glomerulonephritis, and metastatic infection to bones, joints, spleen, or other organs.

The diagnosis of infective endocarditis requires a combination of clinical findings, imaging, and microbiologic evidence. The modified Duke criteria (**Table 1**) are most commonly used to determine the diagnosis of endocarditis. Definite endocarditis is either made by histology or culture of a vegetation or intracardiac abscess OR by

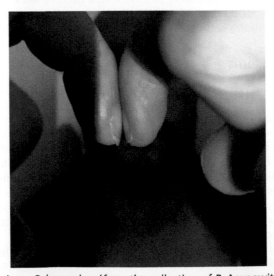

Fig. 4. Janeway lesions, Osler nodes. (*from* the collection of P. Aronowitz)

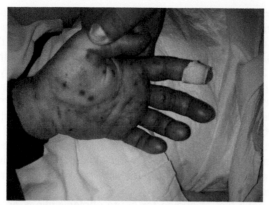

Fig. 5. Petechiae. (*with permission* from the collection of T. Levy)

the following: 2 major criteria OR 1 major and 3 minor OR 5 minor criteria. Possible infective endocarditis is made with 1 major and 1 minor criteria OR 3 minor criteria.[7]

Treatment of infective endocarditis involves prompt initiation of antimicrobial therapy, removal of any infected devices, and monitoring for the need for surgical management. Empiric antibiotics should be started AFTER blood cultures are obtained and should cover staphylococcus aureus (including methicillin-resistant), streptococci, and enterococci. Once culture-specific data are obtained, antibiotics can be tailored to sensitivity results and are generally continued for 4 to 6 weeks. Patients with prosthetic valves may require valve replacement in addition to antibiotics.[7]

ACUTE CHOLECYSTITIS

Cholelithiasis is a common condition affecting 20 million Americans yearly. While most patients with gallstones are asymptomatic, up to 4% per year will develop biliary colic, and 20% of patients with biliary colic will go on to develop acute cholecystitis.[8] In recent years, the rates of acute cholecystitis have decreased as a result of patients opting for elective cholecystectomy for symptomatic gallstones.[9]

The primary symptom of acute cholecystitis starts as biliary colic, which is defined as pain in the right upper quadrant or epigastrium. Pain typically coincides with a stone impacted in the neck of the gallbladder. In acute cholecystitis, this pain persists as inflammation and distension of the gallbladder develop. Anorexia, nausea, and vomiting are other common symptoms during acute cholecystitis.

Table 1 Modified Duke criteria for infective endocarditis	
Major Criteria	Positive Blood Cultures (at least 2 for organisms typically associated with IE; at least 3 for organisms less commonly associated or may be skin contaminant) Evidence of endocardial involvement by: Echocardiographic evidence (vegetation, abscess, or new partial dehiscence of valve) OR New valvular regurgitation
Minor Criteria	Predisposing condition (IVDU or predisposing heart/valve condition) Fever >100.4 Vascular phenomena Immunologic phenomena Microbiologic criteria not meeting major criteria

The physical examination in acute cholecystitis often includes tenderness of the right upper quadrant (RUQ) with or without guarding. Murphy's sign is defined as the sudden arrest of inspiration as the RUQ is palpated while the patient is attempting to inspire and has a sensitivity of 65% and a specificity of 87% with a positive likelihood ratio (LR) of 2.8 and a negative LR of 0.5.[9,10] A fever is variably present in acute cholecystitis. The presence of back tenderness argues against cholecystitis (LR 0.4).[10] The physical examination, specifically the presence of RUQ tenderness or a positive Murphy's sign, is less accurate in the elderly as they may present with acute cholecystitis without any abdominal tenderness.[10,11]

Laboratory evaluation in acute cholecystitis may reveal an elevated white blood cell count. Transaminases, bilirubin, alkaline phosphatase, and C-reactive protein may all be elevated but these findings are neither sensitive nor specific enough to be helpful in the diagnosis of acute cholecystitis.[12]

The initial diagnostic test of choice for acute cholecystitis is an ultrasound of the RUQ. Ultrasonography findings of acute cholecystitis include gallbladder wall thickening, peri-cholecystic fluid, and the presence of sonographic Murphy's sign (pain elicited as the ultrasound probe is pushed against the inflamed gallbladder.) A sonographic Murphy's sign has much better diagnostic accuracy because visualization of the gallbladder is used to determine the precise location of the gallbladder. A sonographic Murphy's sign has a positive LR of 9.9 and a negative LR of 0.4.[10] Ultrasonography detects approximately 95% of cases of acute cholecystitis.[8,12] If the diagnosis is still suspected after a negative ultrasound, hepatobiliary scintigraphy can be performed.[12]

The treatment of choice for acute cholecystitis is early laparoscopic cholecystectomy. Early cholecystectomy has been shown to reduce hospital length of stay as compared with delayed cholecystectomy. Additionally, patients who receive delayed cholecystectomy are at risk for requiring a procedure for persistent or recurrent symptoms before their planned operation.[8] Adjunctive antibiotics are used immediately before the cholecystectomy. If patients cannot undergo early surgery and show signs of systemic infection, the infectious disease society of America (IDSA) recommends systemic antibiotics.[13] Appropriate antimicrobial therapy includes coverage against enteric gram-negative organisms which would consist of either a second or third-generation cephalosporin with metronidazole or a combination of a fluoroquinolone and metronidazole.[13] The addition of Vancomycin should also be considered in patients with life-threatening illness as enterococci are involved in up to 14% of identified organisms in cholecystitis.[14]

SUMMARY AND CLINICS CARE POINTS

- In cellulitis and erysipelas, the diagnosis is made by history and physical examination. For necrotizing fasciitis, the physical examination is suggestive and the diagnosis is made with the aid of adjunctive laboratory and radiologic testing.
- The physical examination in endocarditis most commonly includes fever and a cardiac murmur. Diagnosis requires additional microbiologic and imaging criteria and the use of the modified Duke Criteria is helpful in making the diagnosis of endocarditis.
- In acute cholecystitis, the physical examination is supportive but diagnosis requires imaging by ultrasound. The physical examination may be less sensitive in the elderly in which tenderness may be absent.

DISCLOSURE

The author has nothing to disclose.

REFERENCES

1. Raff AB, Kroshinsky D. Cellulitis: a review. JAMA 2016;316(3):325–37.
2. Stevens DL, Bisno AL, Chambers HF, et al, Infectious Diseases Society of America. Practice guidelines for the diagnosis and management of skin and soft tissue infections: 2014 update by the Infectious Diseases Society of America. Clin Infect Dis 2014;59(2):e10–52.
3. Gunderson CG, Chang JJ. Risk of deep vein thrombosis in patients with cellulitis and erysipelas: a systematic review and meta-analysis. Thromb Res 2013;132(3): 336–40.
4. Stevens DL, Bryant AE. Necrotizing soft-tissue infections. N Engl J Med 2017; 377(23):2253–65.
5. Wong C-H, Khin L-W, Heng K-S, et al. The LRINEC (Laboratory Risk Indicator for Necrotizing Fasciitis) score: a tool for distinguishing necrotizing fasciitis from other soft tissue infections. Crit Care Med 2004;32(7):1535–41.
6. Baddour LM, Wilson WR, Bayer AS, et al. Infective endocarditis in adults: diagnosis, antimicrobial therapy, and management of complications: a scientific statement for healthcare professionals From the American Heart Association. Circulation 2015;132(15):1435–86.
7. Cahill TJ, Prendergast BD. Infective endocarditis. Lancet 2016;387(10021): 882–93.
8. Trowbridge RL, Rutkowski NK, Shojania KG. Does this patient have acute cholecystitis? JAMA 2003;289(1):80–6.
9. Urbach DR, Stukel TA. Rate of elective cholecystectomy and the incidence of severe
10. McGee SR. Evidence based physical diagnosis. 2nd edition. St. Louis (MO): Elsevier; 2007.
11. Adedeji OA, McAdam WA. Murphy's sign, acute cholecystitis and elderly people. J R Coll Surg Edinb 1996;41(2):88–9.
12. Singer AJ, McCracken G, Henry MC, et al. Correlation among clinical, laboratory, and hepatobiliary scanning findings in patients with suspected acute cholecystitis. Ann Emerg Med 1996;28(3):267–72.
13. Solomkin JS, Mazuski JE, Bradley JS, et al. Diagnosis and Management of Complicated Intra-abdominal Infection in Adults and Children: Guidelines by the Surgical Infection Society and the Infectious Diseases Society of America. Clin Infect Dis 2010;50(2):133–64.
14. David N. Gilbert, Henry F. Chambers, Michael S. Saag, Anddrew T. Pavia, Helen W. Boucher, Douglas Black, David O. Freedman, Kami Kim, Brian S. Schwartz, The Sanford Guide To Antimicrobial Therapy 2021, 51st Edition, Page 18.

Approach to the Patient with a Murmur

John Landefeld, MD, MS*, Melody Tran-Reina, MD, Mark Henderson, MD, MACP

KEYWORDS

- Cardiac auscultation • Valvular heart disease • Murmurs • Physical examination

KEY POINTS

- The cardiac examination consists of auscultation, visualization, palpation, and special maneuvers, all of which can reveal abnormalities suggestive of valvular heart disease.
- Likelihood ratios, calculated from the sensitivity and specificity of a physical finding (or test result), are useful to adjust one's clinical impression or likelihood of a given diagnosis, providing practical information regarding the need for further evaluation or management.
- The most robust likelihood ratios for the cardiac examination pertain to systolic murmurs, the primary focus of this review.

 Video content accompanies this article at http://www.medical.theclinics.com.

INTRODUCTION

As average life expectancy approaches 80 years in the United States, and exceeds 80 years in many other wealthy countries, the prevalence of valvular heart disease is growing, impacting patient quality of life, functional status, and mortality. Recently, advances in valve replacement and repair for patients with valvular heart disease have led to improvements in outcomes for patients with conditions such as mitral regurgitation and aortic stenosis.[1] The identification of patients who might benefit from these and other treatments often depends on a clinician's ability to evaluate for valvular pathologies through the physical examination. Murmurs are initially classified according to their timing in the cardiac cycle, specifically, systolic or diastolic. As they are most common, systolic murmurs will be the focus of this article. Diastolic murmurs generally indicate important underlying valvular pathology, but there is less evidence supporting the diagnostic utility of the accompanying physical examination findings.

Likelihood Ratios

Interpreting the physical examination findings for valvular heart disease requires a basic understanding of likelihood ratios. Likelihood ratios serve to define the relative

Department of Internal Medicine, UC Davis School of Medicine, 4150 V Street, Suite 2400, Sacramento, CA 95817, USA
* Corresponding author.
E-mail address: jclandefeld@ucdavis.edu

Med Clin N Am 106 (2022) 545–555
https://doi.org/10.1016/j.mcna.2021.12.011
0025-7125/22/© 2022 Elsevier Inc. All rights reserved.

utility of a given physical examination maneuver (or test result) and can be applied in clinical scenarios to determine the likelihood that a patient has (or does not have) a particular valvular pathology.

Likelihood ratios are a function of test sensitivity and specificity. A *positive likelihood ratio* (+LR) can be calculated as follows:

$$+LR = \frac{Sensitivity}{1 - Specificity}$$

A + LR can also be articulated as:*

$$+LR = \frac{The\ probability\ that\ a\ person\ with\ Condition\ A'\ tested\ I^2\ positive\ for\ Condition\ A}{The\ probability\ that\ a\ person\ without\ Condition\ A'\ tested'\ positive\ for\ Condition\ A}$$

$$ie. + LR = \frac{The\ probability\ of\ a\ true\ positive}{The\ probability\ of\ a\ false\ positive}$$

A *negative likelihood ratio* can be calculated as follows:

$$-LR = \frac{1 - Sensitivity}{Specificity}$$

A −LR can also be read as:

$$-LR = \frac{The\ probability\ that\ a\ person\ \textbf{with}\ Condition\ A\ tested\ negative\ for\ Condition\ A}{The\ probability\ that\ a\ person\ \textbf{without}\ Condition\ A\ tested\ negative\ for\ Condition\ A}$$

$$ie. - LR = \frac{The\ probability\ of\ a\ false\ negative}{The\ probability\ of\ a\ true\ negative}$$

An LR close to 1 means that the test result or clinical finding does not appreciably change the likelihood of disease. A +LR informs the clinician how much a positive test result (or the presence of a given clinical finding) changes the probability of a disease. A −LR suggests how much a negative test result (or the absence of a given clinical finding) changes the probability of a disease. In this review, we include physical examination findings with LRs greater than 5 or less than 0.2, because such findings sufficiently impact post-test probabilities as to be clinically useful.

Clinicians can apply physical examination findings with a known likelihood ratio to their pretest probability of disease by using a Fagan nomogram, to thus arrive at a post-test probability (**Fig. 1**).[2] The post-test probability informs further diagnostic and therapeutic planning.

AUSCULTATION IN VALVULAR HEART DISEASE

Auscultation of the heart in a patient with suspected valvular heart disease centers around 4 core components: timing, intensity, onomatopoeia, and location. A precise description of murmurs is fundamental to identifying valvular pathology and informing appropriate next steps.

---

* In the case of a physical exam finding, 'tested' refers to the probability that a person with Condition A has a particular characteristic physical exam finding associated with Condition A.

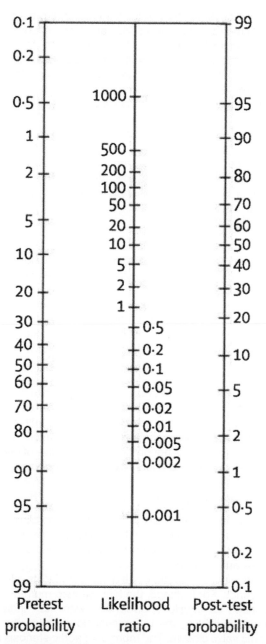

Fig. 1. Fagan nomogram. (*Adapted from* Fagan TJ. Nomogram for Bayes's theorem. N Engl J Med Jul 31, 1975; 293(5):257.)

Timing in the Cardiac Cycle

The first step in classifying a murmur is to characterize its timing. Murmurs may occur in either part of the cardiac cycle (systole or diastole), or in some instances, may be continuous throughout the cycle.

Systolic murmurs, which occur in between the closing of the atrioventricular valves (S1) and the closing of the semilunar valves (S2), are the most common. Diastolic murmurs occur at any time in the longer interval between S2 and S1. One can first identify S1 and S2 by palpating the carotid pulse while auscultating the heart. The heart sound that nearly coincides with the pulse is S1. Systolic murmurs, by far the most common murmurs, should further be described according to when in systole they occur.[3]

Early systolic murmurs: Murmurs with indistinct or obliterated S1 but distinct S2.
Midsystolic murmurs: Murmurs with distinct S1 *and* S2.
Late systolic murmurs: Murmurs with distinct S1 but indistinct or obliterated S2.
Holosystolic murmurs: Murmurs with indistinct or obliterated S1 *and* S2.

Diastolic murmurs tend to occur either immediately after S2, in mid-diastole, or late in diastole (also termed "presystolic"). Early murmurs may obscure S2 and mid-diastolic murmurs (eg, mitral stenosis) often follow an opening *snap* (more on *onomatopoeia* below).

Murmur Intensity

Once the timing of the murmur is established, the examiner should describe its intensity. By convention, intensity is categorized into 6 levels according to the Levine grading system.

Grade 1: Murmurs only audible by listening carefully through the stethoscope for a period of time.
Grade 2: Murmurs audible as soon as the stethoscope is placed on the chest wall.
Grade 3: Murmurs which are loud with the stethoscope but without a palpable thrill.
Grade 4: Murmurs which are loud, still require a stethoscope to be heard, and are associated with a thrill.
Grade 5: Murmurs which are very loud, associated with a thrill, but only require the edge of the stethoscope to contact the chest in order to be heard.
Grade 6: An unusually loud murmur, associated with a thrill, and audible with the stethoscope even when the stethoscope is just off the surface of the chest wall.

The intensity of a murmur alone is not particularly predictive of the underlying cause, but may be useful when considered in context with other findings.

Nature of the Sounds—Onomatopoeia

After determining the timing and intensity of the murmur, the clinician should describe the nature of the murmur. Phonetically imitating aloud the sounds auscultated is a practical way to differentiate various murmurs and to accurately communicate the findings to colleagues and learners.[4]

The clinician should mimic the sound while demonstrating its relationship to the first and second heart sounds. For instance, the high-pitched murmur of mitral regurgitation might be described as "lubHooooooooodub," with "lub" indicating mitral valve closure, "Hooooooooo" indicating the regurgitant flow across the mitral valve, and "dub" indicating aortic valve closure. The murmur of aortic stenosis is often described as "harsh," owing to the combination of both high-pitched and low-pitched sounds. The clinician may hear a guttural "lub gRRRrrr dub" murmur with aortic stenosis. An aortic murmur that has a "blowing" nature is less likely to be severe aortic stenosis (−LR 0.1).[5]

Mitral valve prolapse is a common pathology accompanied by a "midsystolic click" that sounds similar to a "*k*" sound. Regurgitant flow across the mitral valve may develop over time. The combined sound of mitral valve prolapse and mitral regurgitation may be described as "lub...kHooooooooodub."

Sound intensity may also be indicated with onomatopoeia. For example, the early diastolic high frequency blowing decrescendo murmur of aortic regurgitation may obscure S2 and be indicated as "Lub... PEWWww....". If this murmur is grade 3 intensity or louder, the patient likely has moderate to severe aortic regurgitation (+LR 8.2). The absence of the characteristic diastolic murmur is strong evidence against the existence of moderate to severe aortic regurgitation (−LR 0.1).

The low-pitched murmur of mitral stenosis begins in mid-diastole, occasionally after a snap (the sound of the stenotic leaflets opening). It may sound like "up bu duprrrrRR-Rup," with "up" being S1 (which may be louder than normal), "bu" being S2, and "dup" being the opening snap. The rumble may eclipse the beginning of S1.

Location on Chest Wall (Broad or Small Apical-base, Broad Apical, LLSB, Apical Only, Base Only)

The distribution of sound on the chest wall is helpful in differentiating systolic murmurs. The *third left parasternal space* overlies both the aortic and mitral valves and is thus used as a landmark to help classify systolic murmurs into 1 of 6 possible patterns (**Fig. 2**). The primary determinant of a murmur's radiation is *not* necessarily the direction of blood flow, but rather how the abnormal blood flow generates vibrations in the ventricles and/or great arteries, which are also transmitted because of adjacent bony vibration. Vibrations of the ventricles and lower ribs will generate sound *below* the third left parasternal space, and vibrations of the great arteries, sternum, and clavicles will generate sound *above* the third left parasternal space.

The location on the chest wall helps to identify whether murmurs are characteristic for certain valvular pathologies. Increased aortic valve velocity (suggestive of aortic stenosis) results in a broad apical-base pattern (+LR 9.7) on the chest wall. A broad apical pattern increases the probability of mitral regurgitation (+LR 6.8), whereas the left lower sternal pattern increases the probability of tricuspid regurgitation (+LR 8.4).[6]

The diastolic murmur of aortic regurgitation is often heard most prominently at the left sternal border (and occasionally at the right sternal border). The diastolic murmur of pulmonic regurgitation is typically loudest at the left sternal border at the second intercostal space.

All 4 components of auscultation—timing, intensity, onomatopoeia, and location—should be interpreted in relation to one another with their associated likelihood ratios (**Table 1**).

Visualization and Palpation in Valvular Heart Disease

Direct observation of the patient's undraped chest and neck may help determine the etiology of a murmur. Visualization and/or palpation of the cardiac apex may also be helpful; normally there is a single apical impulse per cardiac cycle. A double apical impulse may suggest left ventricular (LV) hypertrophy (+LR 5.6). A hyperkinetic apical impulse may be seen in mitral regurgitation (+LR 11.2). On the other hand, the *absence* of an enlarged apical impulse decreases the probability of moderate to severe aortic regurgitation (−LR 0.1).

With severe tricuspid regurgitation, the right ventricle becomes dilated and occupies the cardiac apex. In systole, the apex may be seen to move inward, and a simultaneous outward motion may be seen at the left or right lower sternal border signifying the increased flow into the dilated right atrium. This visual finding is known as the right ventricular rock (+LR 31.4). A pulsatile liver may also be palpated with severe tricuspid regurgitation (+LR 6.5).[7]

ABOVE AND BELOW THIRD LEFT PARASTERNAL SPACE

Broad apical-base pattern
Murmur extends at least
from the first right parasternal
space to fourth intercostal
space at MCL; may have
diminished intensity at LLSB

Small apical-base pattern
Murmur oriented obliquely
but does not meet criteria
of broad apical-base pattern

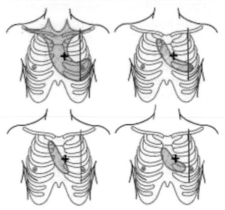

ENTIRELY BELOW THIRD LEFT PARASTERNAL SPACE

Left lower sternal pattern
Murmur along left sternal
edge; may extend to MCL

Broad apical pattern
Murmur in fourth or fifth intercostal
space, or both, and extends at
least from MCL to anterior
axillary line; may extend to
sternum

Isolated apical pattern
Murmur near MCL, fourth or fifth
intercostal space, confined to
diameter of stethoscope

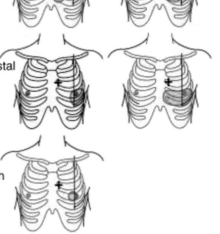

ENTIRELY ABOVE THIRD LEFT PARASTERNAL SPACE

Isolated base pattern
Murmur centered at second
intercostal space or
higher; may radiate to neck
or along clavicles

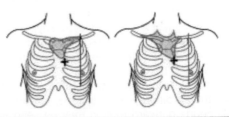

Fig. 2. Location on the chest wall of 6 systolic murmur patterns. (*Reproduced with permission from* Evidence-Based Physical Diagnosis, 4th Ed., Steven McGee, Fig 43.1 Six systolic murmur patterns. Copyright Elsevier 20.)

Table 1
Clinically useful examination findings, as determined by likelihood ratios (+LR > 5, −LR < 0.2)

Finding	Sensitivity (%)	Specificity (%)	Likelihood Ratio if Finding is	
			Present	Absent
Characteristic Systolic Murmur				
Mild tricuspid regurgitation or worse (*LubSHSHSHSHdub in a left-lower sternal pattern*)	23	98	**14.6**	0.8
Mild or worse aortic stenosis (*Lub GRRRR dub in a broad apical-base pattern or small apical-base pattern*)	90	85	**5.9**	**0.1**
Mild or worse mitral regurgitation (*LubSHSHSHSHdub in a broad apical pattern*)	56–75	89–93	**5.4**	0.4
Mitral valve prolapse (*Lub...kSHSHSHdub with midsystolic click in broad apical pattern*)	55	96	**12.1**	0.5
"Blowing" sound throughout aortic flow murmur for significant aortic stenosis	4	67	**0.1**	1.4
Characteristic Diastolic Murmur				
Mild or worse aortic regurgitation (*early diastolic high-frequency decrescendo murmur along lower sternal border*)	54–87	75–98	**9.9**	0.3
Detecting pulmonary regurgitation (*diastolic decrescendo murmur in 2nd intercostal space at left upper sternal border*)	15	99	**17.4**	NS
Intensity of S1 and S2				
S2 inaudible for increased aortic valve peak velocity in aortic stenosis			**12.7**	
Maneuvers				
Louder during inspiration (for TR)	78–95	87–97	**7.8**	**0.2**
Louder with Valsalva strain for HCM	70	95	**14**	0.3
Louder with squat-to-stand (for HCM)	95	84	**6**	**0.1**
Softer with stand-to-squat (for HCM)	88–95	84–97	**7.6**	**0.1**
Softer with passive leg elevation (for HCM)	90	90	**9**	**0.1**
Visualization and Palpation				
Hyperkinetic apical movement (for detecting MR)	74	93	**11.2**	0.3
Double apical movement (for LVH)	57	90	**5.6**	0.5
Right ventricular rock (for TR)	5	100	**31.4**	NS
Pulsatile liver (for TR)	12–30	92–99	**6.5**	NS
C-V wave (for TR)	37	97	**10.9**	0.7

Abbreviation: HCM, hypertrophic cardiomyopathy; LVH, left ventricular hypertrophy; MR, mitral regurgitation; TR, tricuspid regurgitation.

The jugular veins may demonstrate prominent outward pulsations or giant (fused) "c-v" waves in severe tricuspid regurgitation. The x-descent is obliterated and the "v" wave, representing right atrial filling, increases when the regurgitant jet crosses the tricuspid valve from the right ventricle. This finding, also known by the eponym Lancisi sign, can be seen in Video 1 in the online version of this text. It is important to differentiate the jugular venous pulsation from the carotid pulse; bounding carotid arteries may be seen in severe aortic regurgitation.

Patients with aortic regurgitation generate a large stroke volume followed by rapid diastolic emptying of aortic blood into the left ventricle, causing the arterial pulse wave to both rise and collapse abruptly. This is known as water-hammer pulses or Corrigan pulse. The same physiology produces fascinating pulsations throughout the body and has generated many eponyms such as Quincke pulse (capillary pulsations in the nail bed), de Musset sign (bobbing of the head), Müller sign (pulsation of the uvula), and Landolfi sign (pulsatile constriction of the iris, seen in Video 2 in the online version of this text). Although interesting, such findings do not offer particular diagnostic value in terms of likelihood ratios. However, widened pulse pressure (>80 mm Hg) or low diastolic pressure (<50 mm Hg) strongly suggest underlying aortic regurgitation (+LR 10.9 and +LR 19.3, respectively).[8]

By applying these findings on visualization and observation to the findings heard on auscultation, the clinician can further hone the differential diagnosis for a given murmur.

Maneuvers in Valvular Heart Disease

Special maneuvers that change venous return and afterload, can aid the clinician in differentiating the cause of a systolic murmur.

With inspiration, intrathoracic pressure decreases, increasing the volume of blood entering the right-sided chambers from the vena cava, while decreasing return to the left side of the heart. This elevated right-sided volume causes increased flow across the tricuspid and pulmonic valves. A murmur that increases or varies in intensity with inspiration suggests a murmur across the tricuspid or pulmonic valve.

Maneuvers that affect venous return are useful in evaluating suspected hypertrophic cardiomyopathy (HCM), in which the characteristic harsh midsystolic murmur is influenced by the degree of LV outflow tract obstruction by the anterior mitral valve leaflet and the hypertrophic interventricular septum. With the Valsalva maneuver or changing from squatting-to-standing, venous return to the right side of the heart decreases and the LV cavity size diminishes, which aggravates the degree of outflow tract obstruction and thus *increases* the intensity of the murmur (+LR 14 for Valsalva). On the other hand, standing-to-squatting or passive leg elevation both increase venous return, which enlarges the LV cavity size and causes the murmur intensity to decrease (+LR 9 for passive leg elevation). The absence of this characteristic response decreases the probability of HCM (−LR 0.1). Although the greatest risk of sudden death from HCM occurs in patients younger than 30 years, the average age at diagnosis of the condition is increasing (currently at over 50 years).[9] This increasing age likely reflects increased provider awareness and greater use of sensitive imaging modalities. Some of the maneuvers described earlier may be more challenging to conduct in physically limited or frail patients, but the Valsalva maneuver can usually be performed regardless of the patient's functional status.

Proper technique in performing maneuvers such as the Valsalva maneuver is key to eliciting the findings for which you can apply likelihood ratios to aid clinical decisions. The Valsalva maneuver involves expiration against a closed airway for at least 20 seconds. As described by Valsalva, this was accomplished by breathing against a pinched nose and closed mouth. However, this approach can increase pressure in the Eustachian tubes, causing discomfort. Alternatively, breathing out against a closed glottis is a modified technique that may be more tolerable to patients. Patients should be instructed to strain their abdominal muscles as if to rapidly breath out, but to close their mouth and their airway in the back of their throat. To assess whether Valsalva is being performed correctly, the clinician should observe for distended neck veins or facial flushing, and palpate the patient's contracted abdominal muscles. The examiner should listen for a change in the murmur after a 20-second Valsalva strain.

Functional or Innocent Murmurs

Systolic murmurs may be present but without associated valvular pathology by echocardiography. Such murmurs, termed "functional" or "innocent" murmurs based on lack of structural heart disease, are quite common, although their prevalence varies with age. In young adults, the vast majority of systolic murmurs are functional. Although the peak incidence of functional murmurs is around age 3 to 4 years, studies suggest that 86% to 100% of younger adults with a systolic murmur will have a normal echocardiogram. Echocardiograms of elderly patients with systolic murmurs are often normal, although the percentage ranges widely (from 44% to 100%, depending on the study).

Functional murmurs tend to be of lower intensity (usually 2/6 or lower on the Levine grading scale), in early systole or midsystole, and are frequently loudest near the left

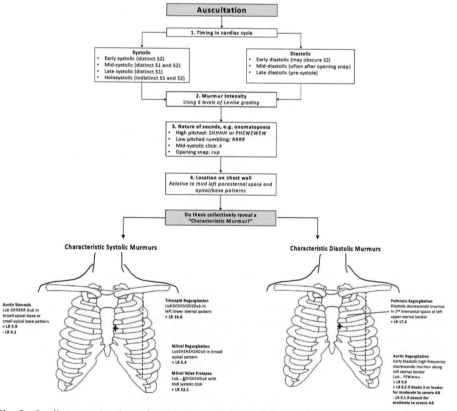

Fig. 3. Cardiac examination of the patient with a murmur.

upper sternal border. Functional murmurs are particularly common in children, and pediatricians have described the *"7 S's"* as key findings suggestive of a functional murmur: sensitive (the murmur changes in intensity with bodily position or respiration), short duration (not holosystolic), single (no clicks or gallops), small (the location is limited or nonradiating), soft (low volume), sweet (not harsh or coarse), and systolic.[10] However, because other pathologic murmurs can also have these characteristics, functional murmurs are defined by the *absence* of other abnormal findings. This includes normal jugular veins, normal apical impulse, normal pulses, no cardiopulmonary symptoms attributable to a pathologic murmur, and a decrease in intensity of the murmur with standing or the Valsalva maneuver.

When a patient has an examination consistent with a functional murmur, the likelihood ratio of the patient having a normal echocardiogram is 4.7. Although not particularly compelling compared with other likelihood ratios discussed in this article, depending on the pretest probability for valvular disease, a clinician could reasonably defer echocardiography in such a patient in accordance with principles of high-value care. It is important to note, however, that functional murmurs may be associated with other high cardiac output disease states (anemia, thyrotoxicosis) that may not present with echocardiographic abnormalities, but may still merit evaluation and treatment.

Putting It Together

After a comprehensive cardiac examination, the clinician can integrate findings to arrive at a differential diagnosis for the murmur in question. This may include the particular valve involved, the direction of flow, and the severity of disease. The flow chart in **Fig. 3** demonstrates one such approach to arriving at likelihood ratios based on these clinical examination results.

CLINICS CARE POINTS

- A systematic approach to the cardiac examination can help determine the cause of a murmur.
- Auscultation forms the crux of the physical examination for patients with murmurs; visualization, palpation, and special maneuvers are useful adjuncts.
- The physical examination is most useful for systolic murmurs, although certain findings strongly suggest aortic regurgitation as the cause of a diastolic murmur.
- Findings with strong likelihood ratios (+LR > 5 or −LR < 0.2) should be applied to the pretest probability to ascertain a post-test probability to inform further evaluation.

SUMMARY

In this article, we presented an exam-based approach to narrowing the differential diagnoses for systolic and diastolic murmurs. The systematic examination of the patient, considering timing, intensity, onomatopoeia, and location of the murmur, as well as visualization, palpation, and special maneuvers, can meaningfully impact the clinician's interpretation of a murmur. Applying likelihood ratios for these findings to the pretest or prior probability of disease allows a prudent, timely, and thoughtful additional diagnostic workup and, in some instances, therapeutic intervention.

DISCLOSURE

The authors have nothing to disclose.

SUPPLEMENTARY DATA

Supplementary data related to this article can be found online at https://doi.org/10.1016/j.mcna.2021.12.011.

REFERENCES

1. Otto CM, Nishimura RA, Bonow RO, et al. 2020 ACC/AHA Guideline for Management of Patients With Valvular Heart Disease: A Report of the American College of Cardiology/American Heart Association Joint Committee on Clinical Practice Guidelines. Circulation 2021;143(5):e72–227.
2. Fagan TJ. Nomogram for Bayes's theorem. N Engl J Med 1975;293(5):257.
3. Etchells E, Bell C, Robb K. Does This Patient Have an Abnormal Systolic Murmur. In: Simel DL, Rennie D, editors. The Rational clinical examination: evidence based clinical diagnosis. New York, (NY): The McGraw-Hill Companies; 2009. p. 433–7.
4. McGee S. Heart Murmurs: General Principles. In: McGee S. The evidence-based physical examination. 3rd edition. Philadelphia, (PA): Elsevier; 2012. p. 351–70.
5. McGee S. Aortic Stenosis. In: McGee S. The evidence-based physical examination. 3rd edition. Philadelphia, (PA): Elsevier; 2012. p. 373–8.
6. McGee S. Etiology and Diagnosis of Systolic Murmurs in Adults. Am J Med 2010; 123(10):913–21.e1.
7. McGee S. Miscellaneous Heart Murmurs. In: McGee S. The evidence-based physical examination. 3rd edition. Philadelphia, (PA): Elsevier; 2012. p. 388–99.
8. Choudhry NK, Etchells EE. Does This Patient Have Aortic Regurgitation. In: Simel DL, Rennie D, editors. The Rational clinical examination: evidence based clinical diagnosis. New York, NY: The McGraw-Hill Companies; 2009. p. 419–27.
9. Canepa M, Fumagalli C, Tini G, et al. Temporal Trend of Age at Diagnosis in Hypertrophic Cardiomyopathy: An Analysis of the International Sarcomeric Human Cardiomyopathy Registry. Circ Heart Fail 2020;13(9):e007230.
10. Bronzetti G, Corzani A. The seven "S" murmurs: an alliteration about innocent murmurs in cardiac auscultation. Clin Pediatr (Phila) 2010;49(7):713.

Moving?

Make sure your subscription moves with you!

To notify us of your new address, find your **Clinics Account Number** (located on your mailing label above your name), and contact customer service at:

Email: journalscustomerservice-usa@elsevier.com

800-654-2452 (subscribers in the U.S. & Canada)
314-447-8871 (subscribers outside of the U.S. & Canada)

Fax number: 314-447-8029

Elsevier Health Sciences Division
Subscription Customer Service
3251 Riverport Lane
Maryland Heights, MO 63043

*To ensure uninterrupted delivery of your subscription, please notify us at least 4 weeks in advance of move.

Printed and bound by CPI Group (UK) Ltd, Croydon, CR0 4YY

03/10/2024

01040471-0013